Trauma Transmission and Sexual Violence

This book grapples with the potential impacts of collective trauma in war-rape survivors' families. Drawing on interethnic and intergenerational participatory action research on reconciliation processes in postconflict Bosnia-Herzegovina, the author examines the risk that female survivors of war-related sexual crimes, now mothers, will breed hatred and further division in the postconflict context. Showing how the historical trauma of sexual abuse among survivors affects the ideas, perceptions, behavioral patterns, and understandings of the ethnic and religious 'Other' or perpetrator, the book also considers the influence of such trauma on other attitudes rarely addressed in peacebuilding programs, such as notions of naturalized gender-based violence, cultural scripts of sexuality, and support for dangerous or violent aspects of the patriarchal social order. It thus seeks to sketch proposals for a curriculum of peacebuilding that takes account of the legacy of war rape in survivors' families and the impact of trauma transmission. As such, *Trauma Transmission and Sexual Violence* will appeal to scholars of politics, sociology, and gender studies with interests in peace and reconciliation processes and war-related sexual violence.

Nena Močnik is a researcher at the CY Cergy-Paris Université, France, and the author of *Sexuality after War Rape: From Narrative to Embodied Research.*

Routledge Research in Gender and Society

For more information about this series, please visit: https://www.routledge.com/
sociology/series/SE0271

Trauma Transmission and Sexual Violence

Reconciliation and Peacebuilding in Postconflict Settings

Nena Močnik

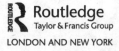

Routledge
Taylor & Francis Group

LONDON AND NEW YORK

First published 2021
by Routledge
2 Park Square, Milton Park, Abingdon, Oxon OX14 4RN

and by Routledge
605 Third Avenue, New York, NY 10017

First issued in paperback 2022

Routledge is an imprint of the Taylor & Francis Group, an informa business

Publisher's Note
The publisher has gone to great lengths to ensure the quality of this
reprint but points out that some imperfections in the original copies may
be apparent.

British Library Cataloguing-in-Publication Data
A catalogue record for this book is available from the British Library

Library of Congress Cataloging-in-Publication Data
A catalog record has been requested for this book

ISBN 13: 978-0-367-53534-6 (pbk)
ISBN 13: 978-0-367-22214-7 (hbk)
ISBN 13: 978-0-429-27379-7 (ebk)

DOI: 10.4324/9780429273797

Typeset in Times New Roman
by Deanta Global Publishing Services, Chennai, India

Contents

Preface

This research is based on ethnographic work in Bosnia-Herzegovina, conducted between 2011 and 2019. It combines data collected from the group interactive workshops, individual conversations, semistructured interviews, spontaneous gatherings, participation with observation, and my own pedagogical practices in prevention of (sexualized) violence.

Throughout the book I refer to mother–survivors simply as 'survivor' if not otherwise stated. In order to minimize the narrative fetishism and to protect people that participated in the research, I provide initials of the first name, sometimes age, and the geographical region. Should the reader require more data or information on ethnographic content, she can contact the author directly.

For the scope of this book, I refer to heteronormative families that consist of a biological mother, father, and children. I do not ignore or deny other forms of families and family relations, nor diverse sexualities and gender spectrum. As my ethnographic work did not include any form other than the one mentioned, I wanted to avoid generalizing or drawing conclusions without any concrete research evidence. However, I hope that this book, despite its limitations, can be a departure point to conduct more research on trauma transmission with all forms and shapes of families in diverse sociopolitical contexts.

1 I will not raise my child to kill your child

Introduction

The beginnings of this book go back to 2015, to a village in central Bosnia-Herzegovina when I was leaving the country after finalizing my previous research. I was visiting women with whom I had worked for half a year to thank them for a fruitful collaboration and the mutual trust, exchanges, and conversations. I traveled with one of them, whom I will call Alma, to a village where another woman that I had worked with, here called Senka, lived with her husband and two daughters. When we arrived, she had just come from the hen house after finishing her morning routine and was changing from her plastic boots to comfortable slippers in front of the house. She warmly invited us to enter, and as is very common in the region, we gathered on a couch, sipping coffee and snacking on wafers. Her husband brought an orangeade from the cellar and then, after briefly shaking our hands, left the house. It was late morning, and the two daughters, aged 13 and 9, were in school. Glancing at the framed pictures of the two girls, Alma expressed how lucky Senka was to have two daughters, while she – although still thankful for her children – had two boys. "They get to help you with your chores, and you have nothing to worry about when you get old as the girls will take care of you," said Alma. "I have worries, more every year," responded Senka. "Every time they are about to return after dawn, I fear they will get attacked. You know how men are here and what they want." This conversation continued back and forth between them, but they never directly addressed their own experiences with men. Yet the shadows of their memories were somehow present in the room.

Signaling that she wanted to get away from the topic, Alma lit another cigarette and, while exhaling, turned to Senka. "I don't know what kind of mother raises her son to go against the woman. You know that I am not raising my boys to hurt, let alone kill, your girls." After a short pause, she added, "Or any girl, ever." It was hard for me to understand if her expression was anger, guilt, blame, or frustration. But it seemed important that she gave her word to Senka to be a mother who would never raise a murderer. Or a rapist.

For a moment, there was a feeling of sudden estrangement, a stop in time. Perhaps there was the realization, a brief reflection of the burden of a survivor, now mother, and her everyday preoccupation with how to prevent the transfer of this burden of trauma, to her offspring. If they were to have met outside of the house, they would perhaps easily agree that they understand each other because they share the same memory of the war, because they both had the same experience. They were both raped. Now, they shared another similar role – that of mother. Yet one was a mother to boys; the other was a mother to girls. What they feared was that one of them would raise victims; the other would raise perpetrators. For both, there was perhaps a sense of responsibility and a feeling that it was all about them, the mothers. Perhaps the onus was on them to raise a generation that would not be haunted by the past but, rather, would learn from their mothers' pasts and never repeat those circumstances in the future. This burden of a responsibility born of their pasts, although mostly uncommunicated in a cognitive way, is real for not only these two women but also for many rape survivors who are now mothers. *What do I tell my kids about my past? How do I share with them my story but keep them from feeling rage? Or disgust for me? Not to shame me or abandon me?*

Despite rich feminist scholarship and widespread pedagogy, in most of the world in the twenty-first century, mothers are still the main pillars raising the family. While giving their best through mothering, many women have to cope with their own traumas in order to spare their descendants the hostile results of intergenerational effects from the trauma transmission. Both Alma and Senka survived captivity, sexual violence, and rape, and, afterward, both were internally displaced. They each remarried and started families but were never able to return to their places of origin.

I had a chance to meet them at their regular occupational therapy group, where they and other survivors meet to knit and spend time together. One of them is receiving financial compensation as an officially recognized survivor; the other is unemployed and still in the process of obtaining this status. In their aspirations for restorative justice, they have both contributed to different state and international institutions by giving their testimonies. Both have collaborated with individual researchers and journalists. In addition, they regularly attend protests, sign petitions, and have been otherwise proactive in giving a voice to the issues of the stigma, public recognition, and social ostracism of women who are war-rape survivors.

Regardless of this activism, mothering is their priority, a part of their life where they feel they have agency. Sometimes, they act as if the lives they led during the war have been frozen in the past for years. It is true that in those frozen years, they were assigned new roles that, in fact, radically changed their life paths and perhaps forever labeled them as survivors of war rape. But becoming a good mother in the aftermath, with the power to teach their kids what they perceived to be good values, useful skills, and vital knowledge about the world, was evidence that a "normal" life had returned. Before the war, many had seen their future in mothering. For those who eventually did become mothers, despite the violent interruption of the war and despite the devastating damage to their sense of self, becoming a mother after the war was a sign of overcoming the past. For some, it was proof of their survival.

Today, Senka and Alma, and many other mothers I have met on my research journey, fully indulge in mothering, keeping their kids and grandkids at the center of their attention with a determined mission to teach them what their mothers taught them – to be not just good humans but also good husbands and wives, and, for their daughters, to become good mothers. What was not expressed as often by those who had sons was raising their boys to be good fathers. More often, they emphasized that they hoped to see their sons become fair and righteous men who do not steal or beat their wives and who do not drink or participate in murky business dealings.

Returning to certain traditional values and lifestyles, taking over the social roles that they are familiar with, is a prevalent trend for many postconflict societies. This return to the familiar not only symbolically denies that the war ever happened but also offers safety and known and predictable life situations. After spending years under chaotic and anarchic circumstances of war, traditional cultural patterns help survivors regain a sense of control over their lives, and this becomes particularly overt through mothering. Most of the mothers in peripheral regions where I conducted the majority of my ethnographic research apply the traditional hegemonic patriarchal rules in their maternal practices. Despite their war rape experiences, they feel that they have to fulfill their duty as mothers, and the role came effortlessly to them soon after the war. For some, motherhood was a revival of sorts, a return to normal. Others believe that it helped them move on and heal. Some did not want to look back and wanted to focus only on the future and the well-being of their children. Still others use the past to spur their resistance – which they pursue for the sake of their children and a better future.

But surprisingly, very few researchers have paid attention to how mother–survivors of war rapes navigate life between their own process of healing from trauma, their struggle for restorative justice, and their role as a mother, especially as it pertains to socialization in terms of gender and sexuality. While the subject of their children continually arose in conversations and encounters I'd had with survivors since the beginning of my research back in 2011, it had only recently occurred to me how deeply their experience of war rape was embedded in their mothering when it came to socialization about gender roles and sexual scripts. Until that very moment when I was listening to Alma and Senka, I had mostly thought of survivors as *survivors*, encompassing how they embraced (or not) the experience of war rape, how they co-created the collective memory, how they established new identities in the aftermath of the war, and how the healing process helped them reintegrate into the broader society. Only rarely had I reflected on the ways each woman's violent past interlaced with the role of mother in the aftermath of the war and the unstable present day of their children and grandchildren.

In the aftermath of the war, motherhood has been recognized in today's collective memory of Bosnia-Herzegovina as mainly (although not exclusively) in two contexts. When referring to mothers, one will most probably first come across the Mothers of Srebrenica, a grassroots movement of mothers searching for their loved ones and demanding the truth about, and recognition of, genocidal crimes perpetrated against their family members, particularly their male family members: sons, husbands, brothers, and fathers. Although testimonies about sexual crimes and violence have also been reported in relation to the Srebrenica massacre, and several scholars have critically examined the abuse of power and sexual exploitation of local women by Dutch UN peace-keepers, the question of rape has been somewhat alienated from the main focus of the group. In fact, I have personally experienced avoidance of this topic when I sought more evidence on war-rape survivors among mothers from Srebrenica. While one of the surviving mothers shared with me her story of being asked for sexual and emotional compensation in exchange for some essential household goods she needed after being internally displaced, she then changed the topic whenever I tried to bring sexual violence and motherhood together in the same conversation.

However, interest has recently begun to increase on a national and international level with regard to mothers who gave birth as a direct consequence of war rape. Those women and the stigma related to this issue came to prominence in great measure because of help from their now adult children, many of whom decided to engage in activist work and speak openly about issues related to the long-term legacy of war rapes. Contrary to the mothers of Srebrenica, who committed their lives to searching for the remains of their lost sons, mothers of children born as a result of war rape have struggled with losing their children by giving them away at birth. In a culture where women can only be fully accomplished through acts of self-sacrificing caring and nurturing, giving away an unwanted child is yet another trauma for the war-rape survivor to carry with her in the aftermath. The struggle of those mothers in accepting the guilt and stigma is constantly reinforced through socially favored myths of ideal motherhood, wherein a mother, the "primal giver of life," subjugates her own needs to those of her offspring. While these traumas are socially inflicted and perpetuated, most of the mothers are left to their own devices to cope with posttraumatic stress disorder (PTSD) symptoms and taking care of their own healing and social reintegration.

Unlike the mothers from Srebrenica, who after years of efforts to gain restorative and retributive justice started to receive recognition, respect, and honorable status in the international community, mothers of children conceived through war rapes remain in the shadows. Other than these two mothering experiences related to the war, little to nothing is said about survivors who became mothers only in years after the war. While they perhaps did not lose their children in combat nor had to decide whether to keep or give away the "perpetrator's" child, they also carry the burden of traumatic experiences of war rape and sexual violence. But all of those mothers, in one way or another, question how to incorporate their war rape experience into mothering in such a way that prevents the transmission of destructive emotions like rage or hatred but, rather, results in their children giving them loving support and safe shelter but also working toward reconciliation and sustaining peace in the aftermaths of the conflict.

A common characteristic in the narratives of mothering experiences from women who were sexually traumatized during the war is their struggle between two seemingly incompatible identities, a *war-rape survivor*, on the one hand, and *a mother*, on the other. Despite these split identities, for many women, mothering has been a crucial step toward embracing healing from the trauma. It has helped many survivors to make sense of the aftermath of the war and provided them with a reason to move on and live again. The decision to focus on mothering after a war rape experience often presents a survival strategy through which one is able also to postpone the systematic and intentional process of healing and coming to terms with the trauma. By being fully occupied with taking care of children, and later, grandchildren, survivors have been able to suppress their experience of rape for many years. For those who suppressed these traumas, *did they succeed in protecting their offspring from potentially transmitted trauma? Did any of the children or grandchildren suspect or feel something in their mother's past and search for more information? Was suppressing the trauma beneficial for the descendant's future?*

Although being haunted by the legacy of rape and facing difficulties in denying their personal history was part of the everyday struggle, most of the survivors I spoke to had never disclosed their experience to their children. In the years immediately following the war, the sociopolitical denial of war rapes was so prevalent that disclosure was impossible. Furthermore, many survivors were preoccupied by the survival of their loved ones first. They were busy with rebuilding, emotionally and physically, their now destroyed world, and, at the same time, they feared stigmatization and being abandoned. Unfortunately, this was what actually happened to some of the survivors who were courageous and trusting enough to hope for the support and understanding of their families. But it happened also to some of the survivors who faithfully believed that silence would help them bury their past and the trauma and live only with their postwar newly attained role of mother. After years had passed, the tool of silence had bounced back and become so defining for their identity that today, although there are more opportunities and better chances for disclosure, some survivors cannot establish their identities and social relationships outside of the social expectation of silent/silenced survivor.

I address this in the very beginning of the book through the prism of "narrated silences," as I believe that this intentionally created and systematically reproduced discursive mechanism attached to the experience of the survivors has had an important influence on the production of knowledge and the representation of survivors that we have today. But in addition, it has influenced how we approach incorporating questions about the legacy of war rape in today's (peace) education. Societal preferences for silence, with the implication that silence is the most dignified position for survivors, has allowed everyone in society, particularly survivors, to confirm that opening up to their children is not going to be beneficial for anyone. Narrated silences help with the reasoning that sharing testimonies with survivors' family members only causes the children to have confused feelings toward their mothers and risks alienation of the mother–child relationship or creates mistrust of maternal authority. In addition, many believe that the silence in fact protects children from the toxic legacies of the violent past. While sharing the story would perhaps ease the survivor's pain, it also risks the pain of becoming owned by their children. At worst, the pain might get turned into revenge fantasies and biases that could lead to intergroup hatred with ethnic profiling based on the roles that the ethnic groups played in the war and the postwar criminal proceedings: those of survivors or of perpetrators.

The narrated silences also explain the paradoxical social statement about war rapes today: while survivors are supposedly silent, the persistent resistance of local and international activists, scholars, artists, and engaged civic populations have made the crime of war rape visible and widely discussed. The rights and political demands of women survivors are being slowly, yet increasingly, met, and there is social progress against denial and stigmatization. The topic is brought to public attention through street protests, events, and public commemorations. For the descendants and postwar generations in general, this means that no matter how strong the intentions originally were to ensure that the silence remained unshattered and unbroken and how persistently these mothers kept their mouths shut, when growing up in today's Bosnia-Herzegovina it is almost impossible to not learn about war rapes and the long-term trauma of survivors. Not only are today's postwar generations exposed to the continuous flow of information on social media but also the developments in memory politics have made active participation much easier and activities related to this topic more accessible. While I believe that children are not merely passive receivers of their parents' collective memory, the ethnographic evidence for how families can contribute in either ideological consumption or critical learning when dealing with violent pasts is still vague and sometimes discrepant.

Despite their different experiences, understandings, and perceptions of surviving war rape, most of the mother–survivors have never been able to fully recover from the trauma, and as a result, the trauma has, despite their efforts to the contrary, become persistently present within their families. No matter how great the joy of seeing children and grandchildren grow and prosper in their lives, the burden of surviving war rape and how to share this with their kids remained. So the stigma attached to survivors of war rape remains and is passed on not only by one survivor to another but also from one generation to another. From the time that girls are born, we are told that we are not safe. You know that you are at risk because of your gender and are taught that it is your sexuality that makes you vulnerable. If most of our mothers told us this because their mothers had told them the same, what do mothers who were not told the same story but experienced it in their own bodies tell us? If our identity as women includes the shared experience of fear of *potential* male inflicted sexual violence, *how do survivors of war rape, who are victims of this in a very immediate sense, incorporate these experiences into their mothering practices? How do survivors for whom justice has never been done and whose attackers have never been prosecuted manage to negotiate their complex emotions, calls for forgiveness, and the nurturing of a positive attitude toward reconciliation?*

The importance of intergenerational dialogue has been widely promoted, but in practice, it is hard to get parents and grandparents on board when they have never had access to effective methods of healing their own traumas. In the case of survivors of war rape, this is made even more difficult due to mothers whose experiences are hidden behind the wall of silence and who have not openly shared their experiences, even with other women who experienced the same trauma or in spaces where they could receive support services. I remember one of the first encounters I had with a group of women when I was presenting the purpose of the research. The leader shut me down, saying, "No woman has ever spoken to their kids, so they have nothing to say in this research." However, with persistence and by posing semi-rhetorical questions, I asked them, "But would you like to share with your kids what happened to you? Do you think this would be something important for you?" After a moment, the silence broke, and I was unable to catch everything they said because the women were talking over each other. It was clear that, in fact, those women *had a lot to say in this research*. There was a need to have space to talk about this, and so we started to meet.

Researching and understanding the impact of these mothers on their children and grandchildren in a cultural context where women still represent one of the most important pillars of the family seems to be of the utmost importance prior to embarking on any efforts toward peace education. Years ago, when I was engaged in various multicultural and peace education programs as a youth worker, I began to question our time-limited impact during the occasional workshops and summer programs in comparison to that of family members and peers who remained in a young person's life long after our educators' intervention was over. Young people would stay in our programs for a week or two as we covered a hyper-energized and optimistic schedule prioritizing peace, tolerance, diversity, and equality. Afterward, they would return to the close-knit environments of their families, schools, and peers. But how sustainable can such youth peace programs be in postconflict zones if we do not consider the threat of trauma transmission in families? While a critical approach to dealing with the ideologically loaded history curricula in the postwar context is now a preoccupation of many educators and scholars, in most cases, family is still the first and most important factor in socialization. It is important for all of us who work in education to learn how to cope with the transmitted, learned, and internalized war legacies that children bring to the schools.

This book grapples with the complex nexus of the potential impacts of collective trauma in war-rape survivors' families in the midst of reconciliation processes in postconflict Bosnia-Herzegovina. With the illustration of ethnographic data, I debate arguments and restraints regarding evidence of risk, whereby survivors of war-related sex crimes who are now mothers might become breeders of hatred and further division in the postconflict context. In the first part of the book, "Social (Ab)uses of War-Related Sexual Trauma," I introduce the idea of narrated silences mentioned earlier as part of the collective memory of survivors and how this has manifested in social realities, values, and relationships. This introduction presents the reader with a further understanding of how, for many survivors, silence has been argued to be a protective mechanism and a conscious act of not telling in order to avoid stigma or vicarious trauma for their family members, especially children. In this way, the silence of survivors becomes a conscious act intended to prevent trauma transmission. However, the mass rapes in Bosnia-Herzegovina are now a public fact, notwithstanding the number of survivors who remain silent. If not directly from their family members, postwar generations can obtain the stories about these events from the media, their peers, and their friends. Thus, narrated silences might operate as a crucial and sometimes the only source of information for those youngsters to access the stories of their parents. As such, they can intervene powerfully in the spheres of informal education and socialization. They not only inform about the past but, more importantly, they imply how to incorporate the lessons and experiences from the past into their existing sets of values, viewpoints, and cultural (sexual) scripts. For this reason, any recreation and/or reproduction of narratives that can communicate the normalization of harmful social relations, dynamics, or processes holds us as creators responsible for fortifying the efforts of critical mediation and the reading of constructed social realities.

The second part of the book, "Mothering with the Trauma of War Rape," shows, as mothers and grandmothers, women remain a primary pillar of the foundation of family and home as they organize daily life and build relationships with children and grandchildren. Despite much excellent work on the psychosocial repercussions of war trauma, displacement, and the postwar mother–child dyad, little is known about how these factors transfer collective memory in terms of continuous hatred and a violent (sexual) culture. Based on these premises, this part of the book looks more closely at the family dynamics of women survivors of war rape and war-related sexual violence and focuses specifically on the potential correlations between child-rearing, trauma, and the transmission of hatred as a response to frustrating postwar injustices. Furthermore, it attempts to answer the question of the impact of a traumatic family past on the children's upbringing, particularly in the understanding of gendered roles and the reestablishment of normative sexuality, which as long as it is based on patriarchy, is arguably inherently violent. I ask, *what effects do feelings of hatred and revenge toward the ethnic other have on boys, and what effect does the display of determined victimhood have on girls/victims, especially the gendered idea of powerlessness, innocence, and shame and, hence, the idea that women are inherently rapable?*

The third part of the book, "Intergenerational Effects of Trauma Transmission and Continuation of Violent Sexual Culture," moves away from the intimate family environment and focuses on wider questions regarding the willingness and urgency to forgive in order to reconcile. Previous research has found the act of forgiveness to be crucial for releasing feelings of anger and revenge toward perpetrators. The act of forgiveness can promote a positive view of reconciliation and lead to postconflict stability; however, the question remains whether real forgiveness is possible before justice is achieved. As those chapters illustrate, most of the survivors continue to fight for justice. At the same time, forgiveness given before perpetrators are prosecuted might lead to further denial as well as forgetting. I reflect on knowledge, emotions, beliefs, and values that second and third generations have potentially internalized, either consciously through conversations or unconsciously through random assumptions and individual searches for information. I attempted to show also how transferring traumatic memory that is derived from war-related sexual violence differs importantly from other war- or genocide-related traumas.

The last part of the book, "War Rape Legacies: Transmission, Agency, Education," presents how different social actors with a specific focus on youth have taken over the processes of the long-term anti-stigmatization of war-rape survivors by incorporating new knowledge and generationally specific narratives on gender, sexuality, and violence. In introducing several projects, I question why specifically peace education in the region today focuses on enhancing interreligious and interethnic dialogues but rarely focuses on identity in relation to sexuality and gender. Furthermore, evidence shows that peace education is not intergenerational when it comes to mother–survivors, as they merely participate in one of the youth programs and almost never let their struggles for justice intersect with the broader field of peace education. This applies as well to the questions related to trauma transmission in families – while it gets addressed as a potential risk and a threat, peace education programs do not really focus on working with mothers and mothering to deal with this.

Before focusing on the main themes of the book, I also wanted to start with a brief reflection on my own voice and methodologies used throughout the ethnographic work. The research approach, ethical concerns, and communication with research participants before, during, and especially after the research, are always my greatest concern. Questioning, adjusting, testing, and evaluating new research approaches has, for me, always been of equal importance as the research theme itself. As I strive to engage more than a traditional researcher, I am always excited to understand the variety of social practices used, for example volunteering with survivors or teaching in summer school with young people in the region, and I see them as an opportunity to reflect on those activities as data collection experiences. Exploring diverse methodologies is, for me, important because I do not think that academic language always translates into fulfilling the immediate needs of research participants. This concrete research, for instance, cannot bring the immediate change that people with whom I collaborate sometimes want in return for their contribution. When you have nothing concrete to offer in return – such as therapy, changes to legislation, the advancing of survivors' rights, or similar actions – it is unreasonable to expect that participants will feel the same level of enthusiasm for participating in a new piece of research as you do. If a survivor has participated since the end of the war in a variety of investigations, reports, networking, and so forth in the belief that life will finally bring her some type of compensation for what she lost and how she suffered, and then finds herself 25 years later still living in the same mostly impoverished circumstances, it is understandable why her first and/or only reaction to a proposed new research project is exhaustion and annoyance. However, I am happy to note that most of the survivors have been motivated to collaborate in this project as they have recognized the importance of incorporating legacies of war-related sexual violence and transmitted traumas from mothers, in peace education, and consequently how with the help of survivors we can develop intergenerational education to break down stigmas related to sexuality and gender and the cycles of historically repeating violence.

For young people, however, talking about a war that happened some ten years before they were born is a double-edged sword. Some of them are very interested in the topic in the sense of avoiding history repeating itself and looking positively to a future of peace and coexistence. These young people attend summer schools and peace education programs to learn ways of promoting reconciliation and social reconstruction. While discourse analysis of the (social) media might show a much less optimistic prognosis for sustained peace in the country, such programs are always an inspiring and motivational force for every peace educator. However, in between these two edges, there is a group of young people who feel indifferent and perceive the topic as irrelevant. They feel this was not their war and, hence, they want nothing to do with it. And I believe this is a fully legitimate and relevant position as any other.

We could learn from the extensive scholarship on trauma transmission in the case of the Holocaust that the third generation becomes particularly vulnerable to the influence of the violent histories of their grandparents, yet I remain puzzled as to whether peace education should help to suppress the pain and trauma of the survivors until they pass away and then construct memories that their descendants will be able to live with, or if we should persist in digging into these personal histories and exploring the kinds of educational and community projects that we should be working on in order to process these emotions and traumas constructively. What kind of pedagogy do we need to develop and employ to ensure that descendants will not be afraid to dig into this long-buried pain but, rather, will accept it as a part of the intergenerational story that we want to learn from but not live again?

This is where my story and my passion come in. I am not a survivor nor a mother. I am writing this book as an educator in the field of humanities and social sciences, with a specific focus on the prevention of (sexualized) violence. Through my teaching, I emphasize the importance of historical legacies in contemporary practices of (sexualized) violence and (gender-based) oppression. Even if they were not directly exposed to war, a student's family history is often reflected in their values, viewpoints, openness, fears, frustrations, and unease. Having the privilege to teach in diverse contexts all around the world, I feel anxious entering a class, knowing that there may always be a student who grew up in a family that suffers from any type of collective trauma. There has been so much collective/political violence and so many mass atrocities in the twentieth and twenty-first centuries that it is almost impossible to be socialized without any reference to the traumatic memory. I was surprised myself in conversations with my father, for instance, himself part of the third post–World War II generation, full of anger and bitterness about current political situations. And I discovered, step-by-step, that it was a reflection of his family traumatic history.

It is not comfortable to commit to the deconstruction of what our students bring to the classroom; it is not comfortable to question the traumatic burdens of our parents and how this (unconsciously) shapes our values, beliefs, and the relationships we establish with others. Despite theoretical and empirical attempts at critical pedagogy, institutional education still avoids perceiving and supporting teaching as a mutual (emotional) exchange that includes unpacking the baggage that we bring into our shared spaces. I believe teaching peace and social coexistence in the isolated, safe space of the classroom, as if there were no memory and heritage attached to it, is not sustainable. I would like to see unpacking happening in my classroom and in the classrooms of my fellow teachers. But before we can do this, we need to have a conversation with those who pack the baggage. I decided to ask mothers first. It was not necessarily the best, let alone easiest way to find these answers, but it certainly took me on an exciting and insightful journey.

2   Edifying ethnography and a voice-in-between

A methodological remark

I recall an event at which I was presenting parts of my previous book, emphasizing in particular the risks and threats to the researcher while engaging with trauma. One of the audience members felt disturbed and asked me why I was making this research a case *about myself* instead of shining a light on the current sociopolitical challenges and obstacles faced by war-rape survivors or any other marginalized group. She argued that research in traumatized settings *should never be* about the researcher's feelings, experiences, and needs, and that talking about myself rather than those who should be my focus – the survivors – was yet another example of why the privileged class, myself included, fails again and again to address the issues of power, oppression, and social justice in general. This feedback came when I had indeed positioned myself at the center of the talk; and I have intentionally attempted to develop the entire paradigm around *myself as a researcher*: *my* emotions, *my* traumatic experience (of vicarious trauma), *my* challenges in addressing the issues methodologically, *my* financial and material obstacles, *my* failure to attract and spark collaboration amongst survivors, and so on. Furthermore, I talked about *my performance*[1], which was not about war rape and survivors' testimonies; again, it was *about myself in the process of research work* with this very topic and my engagements with survivors. To accompany this presentation, I showed pictures *of me* doing all this work.

However, all this *me-me-me* talk was not an egocentric drive to force myself to the front. It was my suggestion to no longer judge the narrative voices in ethnographic research in the hierarchical terms of *whose voice should be heard first, whose voice is real, authentic* or is *more important*. This talk was the outcome of a long, self-reflective process on the very nature of ethnographic research in which – despite one's own ambitions to work toward a more inclusive, balanced, and mutual research approach – the background and social status of the researcher and "the researched" are eventually shown to be unequal. This positioning and balancing have been ongoing processes for me – processes that are as important as any of my theoretical stands and empirical work.

I am not a war (rape) survivor. I am not a mother, nor do I live in a post-conflict setting. What then is the solid ground that legitimizes my voice and absolves my work from taking space and attention away from those who are apparently *voiceless* – the survivors themselves? What gives me the confidence and trustworthy authority to speak on a topic that is apparently so far removed from my own lived experiences? I believe that distinguishing clearly between my identity and my own agenda is what makes my voice in many respects different from the voices of firsthand testimonies. To start with, this project has no ambition of giving a voice to the survivors. For a long time, and especially in recent years, survivors have worked hard to make their own public voices heard. As for the current state of affairs, they have created their own spaces where their voices are loud. Those who want to listen, will hear. There is no need for mediators to provide space or to speak on behalf of survivors. Today, with the help of new media, survivors' stories are omnipresent on the local, national, and international stage. Not all stories have been told; many remain in the shadows. But I would say that there are a sufficient number of stories to help us understand the scope of the crime and its long-term, ongoing consequences. Fear for the "silenced survivors" is rather sensationalistic, but I will address this in the following section of the book.

While plenty of grassroots practitioners and local researchers are doing valuable work in knowledge production, I have found myself in a somehow beneficial *in-between* position – the position of one who might approach the topic from an outsider's view while being well integrated in the insider's world. While an abundance of data has been accumulated, and activities provided by local actors seem to be limitless, all these agendas are also chaotically dispersed and competitively positioned. In theory, collaboration might be beneficial for the sake of visibility and impact, but it becomes financially challenging as funds are limited and hard to obtain. In addition, adopting a grassroots approach to working in a country that is still finding its way to achieving socio, political, and economic stability has its own limitations in terms of target groups and beneficiaries. Working on the ground requires careful navigation when responding to the actual dynamics. However, as an individual researcher I have the freedom and the privilege to find different ways of actively collaborating or to passively follow the work of different local activists, and in this way obtain a broader and more nuanced perspective that they sometimes lack. As I have been returning to the country for several years now, I have engaged myself in different levels of life there – not only professional – I have also built strong friendships. The conversations that I have had within these private relationships have helped me feel closer to the situation in the country than the occasional visitor.

This *in-between position*, I believe, has also led to self-awareness; I am always alert, open, and extremely critical of my own work. Questioning my own voice – which is that of neither a survivor nor a local – is in the end also a strength. "Being one of them" – part of the community that we try to understand – gives one unwritten privilege that one's voice matters the most. While I do agree that the voices of people who live the experience are extremely important, I also want to stay faithful to the basic premises of scientific knowledge which ask us to continuously question our own perspectives, conclusions, and assumptions and to remain open to the new insights and discoveries. Granting unquestioned authenticity to survivors, and fearing accusations of appropriation of their life stories by everyone else, have established dynamics in ethnographic research that impact the way we perceive, use, and work with the testimonies and stories we collect. The vaguely dogmatic postmodern trust in the importance and authenticity of the testimonies of testifiers calls us to review the role of mediators, namely, scholars and writers. As the voice of the voiceless – which very often coincides with the powerless, oppressed, and marginalized – is increasingly reclaimed, the fear of further oppression or the guilt of past sins jeopardizes the need for critical reading and analysis of those stories.

Positioning myself and my voice as mediator at the center is partly a response to this. I assume that research in traumatized settings will always induce certain power relationships and inequalities, if only in terms of access to information, distribution, and diverse audiences. Questioning one's own voice in relation to other voices, positioning the authenticity of the firsthand stories into the writer's own, usually quite different, context, and the hierarchical dynamics of voices, is therefore of the same ethical concern as any other aspect of no-harm policies. When collecting stories from survivors and integrating them in our own research, I argue, we do not misappropriate authenticity or the truth. In fact, combining raw materials from the field with the researcher's own knowledge and experiences produces new narratives that are no less "true" or "authentic" than any other story shared among a particular group of people in a particular context and at a particular time. In a conversation, one survivor tells me:

> Everything that I am telling you here is just how it happened. This is the truth. But now you also have to write about it, but only how it really was, how it all happened (M, Central Bosnia 2017).

For the survivors, the *recognition of truth* is an essential step in healing and therefore in reconciliation. But *the truth* is, as the previous scholarship agreed, often mediated, contextualized, socially constructed. It depends on who you ask, when you ask, where you ask; for therapists, the truth might be the story of the client – a victim; for human rights organizations, truth commissions, and courts, it is victims' stories. For me, the truth in the survivors' testimony is the echo of my own experiences and knowledge; it is also my goal that my research will help to achieve to understand my "truth" better.

Truth, for the survivors, is crucial for collecting evidence and reconstructing the historical and political facts; however, it is also crucial to proceed with the very one-sided, subjective agendas of individuals and collectives. The truth of the violent past is often connected with pain, and pain is not a singular, fixed experience. In a complex event that keeps a society divided – such as a civil war – pain itself may also remain divided. The very process of grasping the truth of the pain is therefore almost always divided too. Lepa Mladjenović (1999, 177) writes:

> my pain is my truth, but your pain is not my truth. If we have a situation in which there are two aggressions, and if my pain and my truth do not give me space for your pain and your truth, can we still create the emotional and cognitive space to hear and care about the Other during two traumatic events that take place at the same time?

The importance of multiperspectivity in violent histories and the ability and necessity to listen, hear, understand, and accept the story and the experience from "the other side" is increasingly acknowledged both in history teaching and in reconciliation studies. However, as experts and as a society, we still lack the effective methodological approaches that would allow us to first collect and provide this multi-sided evidence and then to proceed from there with the action research. In my concrete research, for instance, I have experienced challenges obtaining trust and evidence from groups of women other than Muslims/Bosniaks because my previous work has focused on this community. Furthermore, it is extremely hard emotionally to maintain a balanced multi-perspective approach because "the field" is just not – balanced. I am not referring here to the unfairly popular victim-perpetrator dichotomy but more in terms of access to information and the openness of a community that depends on its very concrete sociopolitical situation at the moment of the research; and also, the general public's approach to the community's own history, which can sometimes be very dispersed and in conflict. Nonetheless, I did not even touch upon questions concerning perpetrators and bystanders, which remains absolutely under addressed. And mostly, I claim, because we have not yet developed a methodology that will enable us to collect the data that will allow us to provide "alternative" perspectives. Therefore, while I theoretically agree with and see the inclusion of a variety of perspectives as crucial in future theoretical and empirical work on restorative justice, I also see the very concrete challenges, obstacles, and dangers in doing so.

Methodological concerns about multiperspectivity yet again intersect with questions of "truth" and "authenticity," and more broadly with the politics of storytelling. Hannah Arendt thinks of storytelling as a vehicle that allows us to expand our understanding and thus to create and sustain plural communities (Arendt 1985, 33). At the same time, she ignores the competing nature of the stories in social politics – not only whose stories will be told and heard, but which will be recognized as true and consequently granted legitimacy by the community (Jackson 2002, 133). Ethnographic work that uses the testimonies of past violent and politicized events enters the field of historical writing in blurred yet important ways that give rise to several other polemics. In *The Dialectics of Unspeakability: Language, Silence and the Narratives of Desubjectifictaion* (1992), Peter Haidu discusses the polemical value of the testimonial narrative in the writing of history, which confronts every historian with at least three challenging tasks: she is to select and organize the material, then present her own level of perspective abstraction and the narrative context in which the collected testimonies will be told (Haidu 1992, 280). As perspectivism is impossible to avoid, Haidu suggests applying "constructivist historiography" in those cases where one conceives of history as a form of writing, "hence as informed by the same structures as all forms of writings" (ibid.). This has recently been widely addressed in memory studies, which in many respects also filled the missing narratives of the very personal, individualized, and one-sided narratives that have long been omitted by traditional historical writings (see Laas 2016; Munslow 2017).

In addition to debates concerning authenticity, previous scholarship also warns of the dangers and risks involved in questioning survivors' stories, and particularly the "authenticity" of those stories (for instance denial, revictimization, etc.). While I might agree on several ethical aspects of such interventions, I also insist on the importance of relational dynamics (Maggio 2014, 92), which include: (1) the process of testifying and storytelling between the storyteller(s) and the listener(s); (2) the roles of individuals and collectives that appear in the stories, no matter if those characters "are real" or have been imagined over the years; (3) the everchanging context and representations of this context; and, finally, (4) how those stories are actively reworked, "both in dialogue with others and within one's own imagination" (Jackson 2002, 15). When storytelling intersects with memory, the stories told tend to involve a component of the imagined histories that serve a desired future: the survivor will tell a story of her past that will help her to achieve her desired future life goals. Very often, these stories are crafted to serve the restorative justice processes, but they also help survivors transit from the position of powerless victims to active survivors. This brings in several different dimensions to understand past events, but can we observe and think of them critically without diminishing "truthfulness" and the "authenticity of the story" as shared by the teller?

In this vein, it is sometimes important to distinguish between the goals of storytelling and story-collecting, which do not necessarily serve the same interest when it comes to the survivor or, more generally, the interlocutor and the researcher. For some survivors, sharing their stories is simply cathartic; for some it is a way of healing, for others a way of surviving; some hope for justice; some hope for compensation. In most cases, survivors do expect *something to happen* if they share their story. It is best if this "something" is concrete and happens soon. Survivors are often particularly motivated to share their testimonies and to collaborate in research when the goal of such projects is to impact restorative and legal justice procedures or to display and distribute data that will, in this or other way, positively impact their lives. It is always challenging to engage survivors when you can only promise them that social change will occur only over a long period of time, becoming perceptible perhaps only in a second or third generation. It is difficult to keep survivors engaged and active when the historical event is receding into the past and when there are few or no changes in their everyday lives. The gap between the number of interviews conducted, evidence collected, and knowledge produced, and the concrete changes that could bring positive benefits to survivors, is frustrating for many. Survivors lose interest in the research when it brings no immediate benefits but only promises of positive change. Not only are "voicing" the crimes and "giving voice" to survivors no longer motivating, but the very nature of how the researcher uses the ethnographic materials does not "voice" only survivors but always also the researcher herself.

This brings us back to the question of authenticity, and more specifically to questions concerning the narrative modes in which we use the newly collected ethnographic materials. The testimony is reproduced "live" in every single inter-action, after which the researcher takes it to another level, cutting it into sections of concrete, real-life illustrations that support her thesis and conceptual framing. I claim that once a researcher decomposes the original story and frames it to fit her own narrative, the ownership of the newly produced meaning becomes shared. Therefore, anything other than a first-person narrative can hardly be called "voic-ing" on behalf or in the name of survivors. Thus, in my research I am "voicing nothing but my own voice," which is without doubt inspired by the storytelling practice and my mutual conversations with survivors.

For example, in Svetlana Alexievich's *The Unwomanly Face of War* (1985), the author, in claiming to give voice to the stories that must be heard, simply collects hundreds of firsthand narratives by women and their experiences of the Second World War. Even in her case, she has clustered and sometimes trimmed entire testimonies to adjust them to the theme and scope of a given chapter. A number of other similar works are also available in the context of the for-mer Yugoslavia.[2] As there is no pretext or interpretation of those source stories, the testimonies mostly remain the ownership of the survivors. In the follow-ing research, the testimonies have been taken from the context of their conduct and repositioned in the new context of the reflecting text. The complexity of the storyteller and her multilayered identity are never introduced to the reader. On the contrary, the excerpts and quotations provided here are rather the reflec-tions of my own thoughts, newly drawn connections and intersections of existing concepts and ontologies, and not the story originally told with a very personal storyteller's narrative and voice.

Increased interest in memory studies reflects a postmodern experience of trauma, in which individuals and communities recognize that there is more to their story than what can be grasped by the official, mainstream narrative. What dis-tinguishes this experience from earlier perspectives on trauma is that people now have a need "for a voice they can recognize as their own; the stories are no longer told by others, by mediators but have their own primary importance" (Frank 2003, 7). The capacity for telling one's own story without mediators has for some time been in the process of being reclaimed. The availability of the means – both lan-guage and the tools for expression – and cultural capital differ widely, but the increase in the amount of space given to the underprivileged and "voiceless" has been tremendous. In this vein, the social status of ethnographic research is chang-ing, and the researcher's role is being radically redefined.

For this research no longer provides evidence *from* the community, *by* the community and *for* the community; it extends beyond these three levels by embracing very different knowledge and experience to provide a theoretical and empirical point of departure for a community, which is not necessarily in any way related – geographically, generationally, socially, or emotionally – to the community where the research is conducted. In sum, this provides the answer to questions about my own motivations in conducting research so far from my symbolical and physical "home": spending a great deal of time in practice as a formal and non-formal educator in (sexualized) violence prevention, questions of recovery, legacy, transmission, and the life in the aftermath of the conflict are crucial.

For me, the value of this particular research lies in the everyday engagement I experience working as an educator both in and outside of the classroom. To discover the motivation to develop new teaching practices and personal approaches in edu-learning environments, and to challenge existing models that might prevent such progress, one needs to better understand the kinds of legacies that leave their mark in our spaces, particularly in what we understand as spaces of trust and safety – our families. Therefore, the stories told by survivors and the voices in which they tell them are essentially different from mine, as are our backgrounds, identities, and our reasons for telling, listening to, and sharing stories. Following the rules of authenticity sometimes ignores the fact that such stories, once written down and published, might be traumatizing for the audience and retraumatizing for survivors. Recontextualization, therefore, provides not only good researcher-designed arguments, but can actually mediate the violent past in a constructive and peace-promoting way. This extends further, offering resistance to fetishistic narratives that still too often fuel orientalist representations, either in portraying the Balkans as the place of "the Other" or the statutes of women in war as victims solely. Unfortunately, I am regularly contacted and invited to join collaborations that would clearly reproduce the toxic and harmful representations against which I devote so much of my work.

My concerns about decontextualization of the stories, questions regarding ownership, voicing, and the constant threat of "othering" and exoticization of survivors resulted in another puzzling methodological question: how much do I want to position this research within the Bosnian experience and how much do I want to think about the questions and themes beyond this geographical and cultural context? Although I am curious about the themes of conflict-related sexual violence, recovery process, restorative justice, victims-perpetrators dynamics, and peace education in a broader, global, theoretical sense, my empirical experiences in other geographical areas are limited. Yet, while conducting the ethnographic part of this research, I have strived to understand the problem through the broader lens of social constructs rather than relying on the local context as geographically unique and historically specific.

It is understandable that survivors perceive their experience as unique and are unable to put it in a perspective that allows them to compare it to other, similar human atrocities. But this is why survivors organize events that center around *their voices*. Not sharing the same experiences allows us, as researchers, to search for lessons applicable to and useful for humanity, which furthermore minimizes the risk of producing orientalist narratives and a hierarchical, uneven distribution of power. In attempting to satisfy the need for authenticity, we fail to address responsibility for specific historic events, cross-culturally and across generations. If the event is so unique, so authentic to one specific context, why would anyone in a completely different context even bother to learn about it? This is how we come to adopt the position of "this cannot happen to me/us" or "this will never happen again." One of my efforts throughout this book, therefore, is an attempt to understand the social dynamics and changes within the limited scope of the case study.

In an educator's mind, educational prevention programs always use concrete cases only for illustrative purposes. It is necessary to leave behind the fetishistic joy of gazing at the suffering of the "Other" and to begin recognizing this "Other" in ourselves. To this end, I have tried as much as possible to avoid referring to concrete individuals with whom I conducted my research. Although some of the materials are extremely interesting and telling, I wanted to consider them as inspiration for my writing rather than materials that would prove my thesis. In the process of research and writing, I have also strived to draw comparisons with the work of fellow researchers in other geographical and sociopolitical contexts as a means to develop an approach whereby my ethnographic practice might inform my edu-learning practice in prevention.

While I am aware of the context and the importance of cultural, social, and political relativism and the uniqueness of every single historical event, I also believe that, in a world that now involves an extensive movement of people and ideas, we must start learning and reapplying culturally specific experiences to the needs of this global exchange. I have tried to limit the amount of firsthand evidence (extracts from interviews), instead bringing in more of the diary notes and observations that I made during my field research work. This corresponds also with my general position of understanding and exploring my own voice and learning processes through ethnographic work, which I can then apply to my practice as educator.

The methodological aspect of grasping experiences that are difficult to grasp even for the informants and then framing those experiences into broad narrative that would simultaneously remain "true" to the individual narratives and protect correspondents who might be at risk as a result of challenging the collective representation, is central to all my writings. For every new project is a new process as well; every writing possesses its own, specific risks of (re)producing the knowledge that perpetuates existing hierarchies, unequal distribution of privilege and power, and the fetishized appropriation that can result from the reconstruction of survivors' vitality and identity in the wake of trauma. Every new encounter with one's interlocutors generates new self-reflections for the researcher, affecting her own impact on the research environments (the spaces of both the interlocutors and the academic/practitioners) and the quest for value in her work. The ethnographer must reconsider the role and the importance of the collected materials, and in what form these materials will be used and referenced once incorporated in the study. This is a particularly demanding task when it comes to following the rigid and strict standards of academic writing. One must also compromise something that contradicts my previous thoughts: namely, in what manner we reduce the complexity of the storyteller's experience, of the event itself and of the entire recovery process.

The value of engaging with and recording conversations with survivors and their family members does not necessarily lie in providing an intellectual understanding of the phenomena investigated from which to propose ultimate conclusions "on behalf" of those from whom one is collecting information. Rather, I see the research process as an opportunity to actively engage with our diverse identities and backgrounds in *mutual exchange* – of experiences, worldviews, and responses to traumatic life events. When the structure of the very investigation is formed as a dialogue it becomes a reflective practice. The very nature of ethnographic practice, which cannot provide a verifiable representation of reality in the complex social laboratory, makes the quest for certainty or tangible conclusions – in the words of philosopher John Dewey – an illusion.

Essentially, ethnographic encounters that include diverse background and identity differences (generational, class, etc.) between the researchers and interlocutors help us to think, visualize, brainstorm, and envision "new worlds." When the research process includes "partners in conversation," the goal of such a relationship does not involve a search for the "truth" or an "authentic voice," nor is the researcher being silenced to give voice to the interlocutors. The value is in the conversation itself, and the very dynamic that enables impactful storytelling at multiple levels, as (1) imagined by the interlocutors before the exchange; (2) told and exchanged in conversation; (3) heard by the researcher; (4) interpreted by the researcher; and (5) read by a reader. And this process never stops; it is infinite and changes every time a new interaction is initiated. For this reason, a *story is the author of people*, as it is not only changed when it is told (Arendt 1985, 50) but is interpreted by the listeners who receive it and determine what to do with it afterward. Why then would the observing and interpreting ethnographer obsessively and anxiously search for the "truth" if she has absolutely no power over this "truth" once it has been handed over to the reader?

To understand the social dimension of trauma transmission in the intergenerational dynamics between war-rape survivors and their offspring, I place the storytelling in my ethnographic practice within the concept of Richard Rorty's (1979) "edifying conversations." To paraphrase Rorty, *edifying ethnography* engages in new, meaningful constructions through interpretations inspired by conversations – not with fellow philosophers, but with informants living, thinking, and reflecting on their experiences in the ethnographic focus. Instead of a question-answer format, the researcher and the research participants in such a practice mutually contribute ideas, feedback, questions, and proposals as to how one might enhance cross-cultural, cross-generational, and cross-political awareness between interconnected social worlds. The diverse backgrounds and identities, privileges, power positions, and social roles of all parties involved in such a practice come to see enrichment rather than obstacles.

As my background training in research methodologies was quite traditional and conservative, I found it crucial to turn toward more flexible methodologies – methodologies that would be engaging; that would still involve firsthand data collection, but which would also provide more legitimate space for my own voice and interpretations, and not necessarily those that are subjected to questions of authenticity and appropriation. Over the course of several years, I have collaborated with the same survivors but was fortunate enough to meet new people along the way. I could follow sociopolitical changes related to the topic and general postconflict development; more importantly, I have seen survivors' lives change, and not always for the better. Nonetheless, as I have grown as a researcher and a woman, I have experienced changes in my own life too. This, of course, affects the very way in which I engage with the survivors today as opposed to five years ago, for instance, as well as it concerns the understanding of the importance of bringing forward my own voice, which resonates with the words and experiences that I have heard from listening to others.

No fixed methodologies might be predicted or anticipated in this constant change and challenge of trying to grasp the knowledge of this very moment, of offering strong conclusions and directions that might create some common ground for further reflection. As a part of knowledge production, the methodological approach is still perceived as a tool which the researcher must define *before* she enters the field. However, to fully embrace the momentum of dynamics, emotions, circumstances, and the micro and macro levels of individuals and communities, the methodological approach must be ever changing. Over time, I learned to leave "my tools" at home, deciding rather to develop my listening skills and to become more attentive and careful, allowing me to navigate more freely, to see the importance of unplanned encounters before scheduled meetings, to be willing and ready to adjust to any moment and to link seemingly unconnected moments into the explanatory stories.

All research is also an exploration of the researcher's own skills, strengths, and weaknesses; it is also an exploration of her role, not only in the research but in the larger social world. While this openness and flexibility might result in more trustful and personal connections amongst the involved parties, this approach also renders the researcher more vulnerable, more "human." Research practice as self-exploration – as a process to enhance one's cognitive abilities and emotional skills – conflicts with the conservative yet governing research standards of objectivity and differentiation from research participants as subjects. But this dehumanized, mechanical type of operation attributes to the researcher not only the ability to observe and analyze a society to which she does not belong; it also assumes that she cannot be affected by the emotional stress and exhaustion which follow active listening and the exchange of traumatic stories.

While the academically approved norms and standards of ethical research conduct are highly structured and regulated, they are often also unrealistic if not artificially enforced. As much as I can theoretically agree that it is important to discuss, learn, and receive training in delivering ethically responsible research, I also have the empirical experience that suggests field work in traumatized settings might often be a wild, chaotic, and dark place. However, there has been little institutional effort in providing researchers with the preparatory self-care training that would ameliorate or prevent emotional fatigue and other psychological fallout, such as secondary trauma. Only after I realized how the trauma from my fieldwork between 2011 and 2015 slowly penetrated all spheres of my private life, impacting it in very negative ways, did I learn that sustainable, fulfilling, and reciprocal ethnographic practice cannot be conducted by a researcher who is psychologically, physically, and emotionally unprepared. In late 2014 and early 2015, when I was wrapping up a long and demanding research work with survivors, I felt exhausted in every way. My sexual life and intimate relationships deteriorated. Hopeless, powerless, and generally unmotivated, I felt resistance to any further work in this field. The risks of becoming traumatized by one's own work had never been introduced at any stage of my studies, my qualitive research training, or while taking the first steps in my academic career. I had to learn it the hard way.

The literature has previously stressed the lack of necessary preparation and training for that undertaking research with traumatized populations (Bell, Kulkani & Dalton 2003; Cunningham 2004; Knight 2010, Bryman 2016). Scholars of field-based social research in particular have emphasized the challenge of design- ing training that can respond to the unpredictability of the processes involved in qualitative research (Dickson-Swift et al. 2008; Coles et al. 2014). Similarly, Amelia van der Merwe and Xanthe Hunt (2019, 16) suggested that ethics applica- tions should include a provision for the proper care of trauma researchers, and that "regular supervision should become a mandatory part of trauma research practice, and if trauma levels are high, the principal researcher may need to invite a trauma counselor to do debriefing" (van der Merwe & Hunt 2019, ibid). Most institu- tions do not currently recognize the complexity and demands of field-based social research in traumatized communities and measure only "tangible" results in the form of publications.

To keep their positions in a competitive academic market, many researchers self-sabotage and deny the signs and symptoms of burnout, emotional fatigue, and vicarious trauma. Individual researchers possess very different capacities and therefore require different levels and layers of self-care, emotional and physical recovery, and recharge in the aftermath of field work. It is therefore crucial to demand and establish an institutional ethos that addresses the fact that researchers can be negatively affected by their work, and that institutions have obligations to present material on indirect trauma (Knight 2013, 238) and to provide systems of prevention and support (van der Merwe & Hunt 2019, 16). One of these systems could involve instruction in self-care methods and well-being strategies. "Turning away," as explained by Karen Saakvitne (2002, 448), refers to making use of individual and institutional tools to make oneself aware of how to prevent and cope with vicarious trauma, with the main goal for researchers being the ability to leave "the relationship once the research is complete" (Dickson-Swift et al. 2006).

However, beyond such direct interventions to protect the physical and mental well-being of researchers, there is another more complex angle to research practice that becomes particularly apparent once *empathetic witnessing* is replaced by *compassionate engagement* – namely, when a researcher, influenced by the political implications of witnessing traumatic stories, begins to feel the need to intervene.

In *Notes from the Field: The Negotiation of Boundaries: Anthropological Clichés, Witnessing and Honest Self-Work*, Karin Friederic (2010, 86) reflected on her own attempt to negotiate the boundaries between *self-as-anthropologist, self-as-activist* and *self-as-friend/participant* in terms of identifying the form of strategic self-work most beneficial to working for social change.

The transition from observational data collection to the critical necessity of applying this data empirically can jeopardize research ethics and may even put the researcher at risk of becoming overwhelmed by the demands and needs of the field. In my own practice, the urge to engage as an activist was also the turning point that led to a deeper connection with my research participants, absorbing their stories and their suffering and consequently experiencing vicarious traumatization. In addition to the critical self-assessment of our skills, emotional and cognitive capacities, and potential personal connections (in terms of our own traumatic histories), as researchers we must therefore seriously define and evaluate our role and, related to this, the goals of our research. Setting realistic boundaries without feeling guilty or powerless and being able to turn away when the work becomes too overwhelming are probably the hardest and most challenging parts of preventive training and preparation. If these boundaries are defined prior to going into the field, self-care strategies and incorporating well-being in everyday life will become much easier and spontaneous practice.

Therefore, excluding oneself from the research practice to ensure objectivity not only presumes that a researcher can put herself "above" the world and automatically establish the hierarchical relationship; it also asks the researcher to enter into the research practice only cognitively. That is, she is required to leave outside her body and her emotional and sensitive experiences of the world. While I believe that some individuals are able to control how well they function in such or other engagements, I do not want to comply with such detachment. The ethnographer who does not invest in her own personal growth, developing her emotional intelligence and strengthening her cognitive skills, will eventually fail to engage in mutually satisfying conversations, and in the long run, harm her own well-being and the well-being of those around her.

In time, my experience of vicarious traumatization raised my own awareness and the need to initiate trainings, workshops, and writing opportunities for those fellow researchers who, between academic engagements and community work, wear multiple hats, and are exposed to suffer from the trauma in relation to this work. Perhaps unsurprisingly, my suggestions were well received by a vast number of co-fellows who had been searching for the tools and support to establish safe research spaces and well-being routines in post-research recovery.[3] Together, we had a chance to share and discuss the tools we all need to embark on their fieldwork research with the confidence and self-esteem of a professional – that is, well equipped, well prepared, and with clear guidance as to how to conduct ethically responsible research while at the same time taking care of our own well-being. For many of the researchers working in the field of trauma, the research process is also a self-investigatory journey. A researcher who has been exposed to trauma is therefore always on a twofold mission: the first is their primary research topic and the second is the exploration of their own perception of the emotions, morally questionable situations, and risky actions they may encounter. Even if it is done in a more or less haphazard way, researchers must make use of their best capacities, skills, and resources – in their own unique manner – to reach out for the information and support that will help them identify possibilities for replenishing their well-being and practicing self-care when their research is completed.

This book, therefore, is not only an attempt to grasp the complex interconnections between intergenerational trauma transmissions from traumatized mothers and the legacy of sexual violence in socialization and peace education, but a reflective practice on existing power dynamics in ethnographic work, a discussion concerning the possibilities of deconstructing or re-establishing new orders and, most importantly, an attempt to understand how to use the outcomes of the ethnographic research to think on and develop pedagogical methods to teach about violent histories. So, bringing the past of some other people, *survivors*, into the present of us, who are merely witnesses, for experiences and rehabilitation to become knowledge and prevention. While rethinking standard ethical concerns involving research participants is an obligatory and indisputable step when embarking upon research, I have paid more attention to what, in my view, remains marginalized: our own growth, challenges, and struggles. The centering of my voice is justified because I am writing not only as a researcher but also as an educator in the prevention of (sexualized) violence. My ethnographic work therefore informs my edu-learning practice. Being an effective edu-learner means also knowing our own (traumatic) histories and learning where the students and/or other learners are coming from: understanding their homes and those who nurture, raise, and socialize them in these homes. In most of the world, the first educators are still the mothers.

Notes

1 In 2015 I created a performance titled "Canned" to cope with the vicarious trauma and the burden of my own privilege(s) while working with survivors. More about the performance was published in "(Un)canning the victims: Embodied research practice and ethnodrama in response to war-rape legacy in Bosnia-Herzegovina." *Liminalities: A Journal of Performance Studies* 14(3): 23–39, 2018.
2 Among which, for instance: *They would never hurt a fly* (2004) by Slavenka Drakulič, or *This was not our war: Bosnian women reclaiming peace* (2004) by Swanee Hunt.
3 In 2018, I initiated the workshop "The Cost of Bearing Witness: Secondary Trauma and Self-Care in Fieldwork-Based Social Research" at the University of Turku, Finland. In 2020 we published a special issue of *Social Epistemologies* under the same title. The issue includes several papers that bring forward various experiences from social researchers in the field and includes their own practices when coping with secondary trauma.

Bibliography

Arendt, H. 1985. *The human condition*. Chicago: University of Chicago Press.
Bell, H., Kulkani, S., and Dalton, L. 2003. "Organizational prevention of vicarious traumatization." *Families in Society* 84 (4): 463–470.

Bryman, A. 2016. *Social research methods*. 5th ed. New York: Oxford University Press.

Coles, J., Astbury, J., Dartnall, E., and Limjerwala, S. 2014. "Qualitative exploration of researcher trauma and researchers' responses to investigating sexual violence." *Violence Against Women* 20 (1): 95–117.

Cunningham, M. 2004. "Avoiding vicarious traumatization: Support, spirituality, and self-care." In N. Boyd Webb (Ed.), *Mass trauma and violence: Helping families and children cope* (327–346). New York: Guilford Press.

Dickson-Swift, V., James, E. L., and Liamputtong, P. (Eds.). 2008. *Undertaking sensitive research in the health and social sciences: Managing boundaries, emotions, and risks*. Cambridge, UK: Cambridge University Press.

Frank, W. A. 1995. *The wounded storyteller: Body illness and ethics*. Chicago: University of Chicago Press.

Friederic, K. 2010. "Notes from the field: The negotiation of boundaries: Anthropological clichés, witnessing and honest self-work." *Arizona Anthropologist* 20: 81–88.

Haidu, P. 1992. "The dialectics of unspeakability: Language, silence and the narratives of desubjectifictaion." In S. Friedlander (Ed.), *Probing the limits of representation: Nazism and the "final solution"* (277–299). Cambridge, MA: Harvard University Press.

Jackson, M. 2002. *The politics of storytelling: Violence, transgression, and intersubjectivity*. Copenhagen: Museum Tusculanum Press.

Knight, C. 2010. "Indirect trauma in the field practicum: Secondary traumatic stress, vicarious trauma, and compassion fatigue among social work students and their field instructors." *Journal of Baccalaureate Social Work* 15 (1): 31–52.

Knight, C. 2013. "Indirect trauma: Implications for self-care, supervision, the organization, and the academic institution." *The Clinical Supervisor* 32 (2): 224–243.

Laas, O. 2016. Toward truthlikeness in historiography. *European Journal of Pragmatism and the Writing of History* 8 (2): 1–29.

Maggio, R. 2014. The anthropology of storytelling and the storytelling of anthropology. *Journal of Comparative Research in Anthropology and Sociology* 5 (2): 89–106.

Mladjenović, L. 1999. "Caring at the same time: On Feminist politics during the NATO bombing of the Federal Republic of Yugoslavia and ethnic cleansing of Albanians in Kosovo." In S. Meintjes (Ed.), *The aftermath: Women in post-conflict transformation* (172–183). London: Zed Books.

Munslow, A. 2017. "History, skepticism and the past." *Rethinking History* 21 (4): 474–488.

Rorty, R. 1979. *Philosophy and the mirror of nature*. Princeton: Princeton University Press.

Saakvitne, K. V. 2002. "Shared trauma: The therapist's increased vulnerability." *Psychoanalytic Dialogues* 12 (3): 443–449.

van der Merwe, A. and Hunt, X. 2019. "Secondary trauma among trauma researchers: Lessons from the field." *Psychological Trauma: Theory, Research, Practice, and Policy* 11 (1): 10–18.

3　Social (ab)uses of war-related sexual trauma

Survivor-centered trauma healing as institutional inhibition to social recovery

I have been sitting in a living room with a survivor I have known now for almost six years. I have only visited her home once before, when I dropped her off in front of her house and waved to her husband, who was picking plums in the garden. This time he was in the kitchen when I arrived, and he joined us in the beginning for coffee and some rather polite small talk. He knows about my work with survivors and the workshops his wife is attending. Before leaving, he starts to tell me that the problem among women survivors is that they "think and talk about the war too much." Afterward, I summed our conversation in my diary:

> Men are damaged very badly. He said he and his colleagues suffer. But the problem with women is that they talk too much. He asked me if I think that it is only women who are traumatized. Men are traumatized even more, because no one talks about men, he said. Men were killing and shooting (he didn't mentioned rapes or anything like this). He sees women attending "therapies" as a problem because in therapy women just bring up their trauma again and again and are never able to close this chapter of their life. I asked him if he sees a solution in the silence and he responded that there is no point in talking when you know you can't change the situation, let alone the past. War has happened and you can't rewind it, he said couple of times, you have to accept it and live with it. I also asked him if he thinks that men manage to work through their traumas if they don't talk, and he said no, he thinks of war every day, and he thinks that other men do as well. But he also thinks that this means they must talk about it or re-think the events again and again. He was rather pessimistic about everything. I didn't feel him to be apathetic though.
>
> (2018)

After he left, his wife added that she knows that he suffers but that he does not want to talk about anything related to the war. We then change the conversation and start to talk about her kids, but she returns to him later, saying:

> Sometimes I want him to listen to me. I don't want to speak about rape, I think I am over this. But I want to tell him that I am not feeling well, you know, sometimes you wake up, and it is raining, and my hip hurts me, and I see no point in anything. And I want to whine, yes, maybe I don't even want to talk about the war, really. I just want to whine, but immediately when I mention war, he tries to stop me, and I just want him to talk to me, do you understand me? Like, comforting me in some way, and maybe to whine with me.
>
> (M52, Central Bosnia 2018)

Other survivors find similar "comfort" in the sharing circles of other survivors. They simply lack someone in their closest circles – either family members or close friends – who would be sensitive enough to listen and therefore to participate in the struggle. The listener must feel the teller's victories, defeats, and silences, "know them from within" (Felman & Laub 1991, 58); listening is always relational, which means that it is not only the teller who re-lives the same experience again; the telling is also traumatic to the listener. The "silences" practiced at home are therefore not necessarily the result of a fear of being abandoned or shamed. When Felman and Laub write that tellers at some level prefer silence "so as to protect themselves from the fear of *being listened to* – and *of listening to themselves*" (ibid.), they might as well decide not to share simply because they believe that the listener has no capacity to respond in a way that would be confirming and comforting.

Many survivors would confirm that being unable to speak about their experiences at home is not rare, and that joining a support group is to a large extent a result of the need to reach out to those who will or can listen and hear. Testimony-based studies conducted soon after the war (Seifert 1994; Allen 1996; Vranić 1996) include cases in which war-rape survivors were abandoned by their husbands or shamed by their family after the disclosure, while other studies show how silence became a long-term solution to the fear of abandonment or ostracism (Lončar et al. 2006; Husić et al. 2014; Delić & Avdibegović 2016). During my fieldwork, this fear was expressed by most of the interlocutors; only a few survivors talked openly about their past with both their husbands and children and felt fully supported by them in all their needs.

However, silence and silencing are, like any other processes, dynamic. I was in conversation with a survivor who told me that her three adult children abandoned her when she first disclosed her experience in 1996. Nonetheless, today she has reestablished and normalized her relationship with them and also has a loving and supporting relationship with her grandchildren. In our conversation, she explained that they never again spoke about this matter after her children's return (although she very much wanted to). Today she understands that their reaction was an impulsive response that most probably came from the shock of hearing the story (field notes, Northeast Bosnia 2018). As a consequence of being abandoned, she has been *dealing with* traumatic symptoms such as depression, physical pain, anxiety, and self-stigmatization. Today, she says that she has managed to come to terms with what happened to her; she feels safe and empowered among other survivors in the organization that she joined in 2015. However, her children have also *dealt with* their mother's concerns and have come to the point where they are able to return to her and accept her *as she is today* and not judge her for the events from her past.

This example tells us much about how strongly the dynamics of silence are attached to the stigma and the process of individual and social recovery of survivors. Talking about silence inevitably links it to the process of (self-)stigmatization and a consideration of the time span required for the individual and social recovery processes of survivors and the postconflict society. For I will argue in the next chapter that "narrated silences" have significantly influenced the nature of the recovery in the aftermath of the war – this has been centered around individual (psycho-) approaches to trauma healing rather than collective (socio)therapy, which has unfortunately also contributed to a culture of impunity as opposed to a culture of accountability when it comes to dealing with crimes and perpetrators.

Following the war-inflicted rapes in Bosnia-Herzegovina, dealing with stigma has usually gone hand in hand with other questions concerning the healing process (Skjelsbaek 2006; Clark 2016; Berry 2017). Although the concept of stigma has its epistemological origin in sociological research, the issues of resilience and – in the case of war-rape survivors – breaking the stigma have taken center stage in therapeutic recovery practices (Lončar et al. 2006; Husić et al. 2014; Funk & Good 2017; also see Pilgrim & McCranie 2013). Psychotherapeutic support that has focused on the stigma experienced by women survivors struggling with PTSD has helped considerably with symptoms such as depression, anxiety, and flashbacks; however, it has also marginalized the entire social aspect of stigma, negatively affecting the successful integration of survivors back into their communities (Davies 2017). Rather than breaking the stigma, the focus on psychological treatment for war-rape survivors has helped promote socio-politically induced crime as a type of mental illness, reinforced rape myths, and promoted a rape culture (e.g., Gavey 2005). In his broad argumentation about stigma and its relation to mental health, William Davies (2017) argues that the "idea that one is simply 'unwell' might provide comfort to people wrestling with their own depression or anxiety"; however, this is the very approach that pushes war-inflicted rape victims to the margins of the fundamentally cultural, political, and economic structures which spread the feeling of being "unwell."

If we understand that the stigmatization of war-rape survivors derives from pre-existing rape myths – that is, "prejudicial, stereotyped, or false beliefs about rape, rape victims, and rapists in creating a climate hostile to rape victims" (Burt 1980, 217) – then the medicalization of trauma related to war rapes holds survivors responsible for their own recovery. If a female survivor does not find the requisite strength to speak out, disclose her agony, and search for help, *she* is to be blamed; yet when she does speak up, this hardly guarantees that the public will recognize the wrongdoings of the perpetrators. Rather, her story tells us about the "strength" of the victim and her "successful" transition from victim to survivor. The act of speaking up has, therefore, become an act of assumed empowerment; it praises the individual and the courageous acts of survivors rather than generating a collective pressure for the legal persecution and punishment of perpetrators.

Whether survivors speak up and risk shattering their social status or remain silent for various reasons, the pressure of speaking up and searching for psychological and medical support serves to establish a common understanding of *where* the responsibility lies (Sayce 1998) – in the survivors themselves. If anything is to be done in regard to justice, *survivors* must be in charge. In this way, treatment and support for the survivors happen in somehow "isolated spaces," mostly in the community (health) centers that offer psychosocial and medical support, where women with the "same experience" can meet, share, and exchange the luxury of being listened to, feeling safe, and feeling relieved. Nonetheless, with limited cooperation from the "outside world" and the wider society, the medical and psychotherapeutic treatment of war-related traumas inflict self-stigmatization, which manifests itself in feelings of shame, embarrassment, and degradation.

The opportunity for psychotherapeutic support and (at one point) financial compensation has been a strong call for survivors to speak out and disclose their war-inflicted rape experiences. At the same time, they have also been offered the safety of a limited, trusted circle of like-minded individuals, creating for some a life "in between" – a concealable stigmatized identity (Smart & Wegner 1998; Quinn & Chaudoir 2009). However, survivors continuously experience the anxiety of being discovered or having to make daily decisions concerning the disclosure of one's story outside the trusted circles – in one's family or community. While having never fully opened up, survivors have internalized the societal belief about the connotation and stigma associated with war-rape survivors (Quinn & Chaudoir 2009).

In 2015, the United Nations Population Fund (hereafter referred to as UNFPA) published the following research: *Stigma Against Survivors of Conflict-Related Sexual Violence in Bosnia-Herzegovina* (UNFPA 2016), which contained qualitative data from 30 survivors of conflict-related sexual violence and quantitative data from a sample of 1,000 randomly selected respondents who were asked to share their opinions about the stigmatization of rape survivors. The main goal of the research was to define the current forms, causes, and perceptions of survivors of conflict-related sexual violence and the marginalizing acts that these individuals face in their everyday lives. Whereas pity, followed by compassion, understanding, and the need for support are the general public's most common reactions, the results from the qualitative research involving 30 survivors show that nearly all of them mentioned self-stigma. Regardless of whether or not their families and community members were aware of their experiences, feelings of shame and guilt prevented them from disclosing them (UNFPA 2016, 4).

The interviews also revealed that two-thirds of the women had been subjected to verbal abuse, condemnation, insults, and humiliation when their experiences were disclosed to the community (UNFPA 2016, 6). Whereas women are more likely to speak freely to family members who survived the war, they tend to fear their children's reaction; the "burden of the secret" and how and/or when to disclose their story to their children remain the concern of many. In a study of the impact of psychological health and well-being on people living with a concealable stigmatized identity, Quinn and Chaudoir (2009) state that the more individuals believe that others will label them according to the associated stigmas, the more symptoms of illness they will experience. This leads inevitably to self-exclusion from the community, "when survivors give credence to the feeling of shame and guilt on which community insists" (UNFPA 2015, 3). When survivors decide to speak up, they are aware and "ready" to accept the "tag" or the designation that comes along with it.

To shift responsibility from survivors to the broader society, Liz Sayce (1998) recommended replacing the term "stigma" with "discrimination" and focusing attention on those *who produce stigma* vis-à-vis the recipients of those behaviors. Similar discursive propositions have come from scholars and practitioners working with rape survivors, suggesting that "victim" be changed to "survivor" to connote agency and control rather than powerlessness and despair (Hesford 1999; Barry 1979; Kelly 1988). While trauma survivors clearly need medical and psychotherapeutic support, the act of positioning individuals in closed social circles will divide them into a distinct category, "a rape survivor," thus accomplishing the separation of "us" and "them." It is obviously extremely difficult to overcome this separation; however, what should be taken into consideration is that working with survivors and the wider community simultaneously could potentially narrow the huge gap that has been created over the years. In their testimonies, survivors often provide concrete examples of situations where they were not being judged or subjected only to stereotypes and prejudices.

When a survivor is abandoned or threatened by their family and/or environment (UNFPA 2016, 6–8, 14) or denied a service (UNFPA 2016, 17) because of their war-inflicted rape experience, we should no longer talk about perceptions but acts – that is, discrimination. While discrimination and stigmatization are crucially interconnected, the psychotherapeutic focus on survivors' well-being fails to stress the lack of privileges they face in their everyday lives with regard to housing, marital status, access to medical treatment, reentry into the job market, and so on. The "disclosure" process for women is full of risk for social repercussions (such as abandonment by the community) when considerable credit is given to the psychological benefits of "speaking out." While this can grant provisional relief, the ensuing social repercussions may cause severe retraumatization and exacerbate the symptoms of PTSD.

When we talk about "legacies" and how the experiences of survivors – now mothers – can leave potentially harmful traces in their family, it is not enough to address silence and stigma(tization) through psychotherapeutic and individual prisms. I claim that the importance of transforming society into an environment conducive to healing survivors has been almost completely ignored for the last two decades. Looking toward "socio-" rather than "psycho-" therapy would significantly shift society's understanding of survivors' social status and mental health from their own individual intrapsychological imbalances and struggles to being the consequences of different sociopolitical factors. Given the prevalence of individualism and the view of the "self" as the nucleus in most of today's Western-influenced societies, the importance and healing potential of sociotherapy have been overshadowed by psychotherapy.

The sociotherapy approach strives to conduct therapeutic activity from a sociological perspective (Akman 2015, 10), in which an individual is not a dissociated member of society. Stuart Whitely (1986, 721) emphasizes that, compared to psychotherapy – which is primarily a *listening* process – sociotherapy necessitates *interaction*; it encourages the development of more efficient coping strategies for interpersonal interactions. The therapeutic effect derives from the active input of the group members as they participate, question, advise, influence, and correct each other in their social contact (Richters et al. 2010, 99). When the direct psychological and physiological traumatic symptoms (e.g., PTSD, depression, and anxiety) and self-stigmatization of war-rape survivors are approached within the context of intrapersonal systems – which are central to the psychotherapeutic approach – stigma-power illustrates the need for social, cultural, political, and hence sociotherapeutic approaches to healing the trauma of war-rape survivors (Edelson 1970, 176).

Treating the symptoms of PTSD solely within psychotherapeutic practice subtly denies acknowledging war rapes as socio-politically created weapons of war. To a certain degree, the group therapies offered by NGOs and grassroots survivors' organizations, which structure their work around group sharing or group testifying, have taken this aspect into consideration by applying some of the principles of sociotherapy. This can be observed most visibly in attempts to break down victimized identities and replace them with the seemingly more empowering identity of "survivors." Common sociotherapeutic methods strive to help survivors regain their self-respect and to value their individual input against self-stigmatization, raising hope and instilling trust into society, overcoming self-blame, and exercising forgiveness (Richters et al. 2010, 105).

However, there is a high risk that the idea of the sociotherapy will be misused, particularly when it comes to stigma and stigma-power. It can be particularly risky when it includes only survivors. In traditional approaches to sociotherapy, the main responsibility for social change lies with the individual's own actions and shifts in behavior patterns, attitudes, and perceptions. In contrast to psychotherapy, individuals in sociotherapy analyze their struggles through introspection but also strive to develop new behaviors and attitudes in order to cope with external challenges. Considering the elements of sociotherapy as a departure point, I propose extending the understanding of "socio" and "therapy" into the existing practice of psychotherapy. While survivors can commit themselves to the notion that, for instance, society can change, improve, accept them and their stories, and help them find the strength to share their stories, sociotherapy should reconsider the active participation of the social members with whom survivors intend to establish a relationship (e.g., with family members who shame and blame them for being raped).

Hence, self-stigmatization (individually inflicted action), for example, is a consequence of external social pressure but can be approached and healed through sociotherapy. On the other hand, stigmatization (socially inflicted actions such as stereotypes, prejudices, and discrimination) cannot be tackled simply by survivors changing their behavior, attitudes, and perceptions when others do not. Stigma is a social process that demands the "relearning of social roles and interpersonal behavior through the experiencing of social interactions in a corrective environment" (Whiteley 1986, 721) or resocialization of the established problematic values and behaviors learned from the surrounding social environment (e.g. school, family, friends, etc.) (in Kannenberg 2003, 90). For survivors to "unlearn" self-stigmatization and for members of their community to "unlearn" stigmatization, it is crucial to examine the motives and interests of those individuals or their social groups attained through stigmatization. Specifically, it is imperative to consider the power of stigma and how certain individuals benefit when others are shamed and shunned.

Phelan et al. (2008) identify several advantages from which individuals or social groups can benefit by perpetuating stigma. *Keeping some people down*, the first advantage, cumulates wealth, power, and high social status for others. The second advantage, *keeping people in*, allows one to distinguish "us" from "them," constructing rules that regulate, navigate, and control peoples' everyday behavior and social (inter)actions to avoid chaos, anarchy, and resistance. In the third advantage, *keeping people away*, stigma separates the healthy from the unhealthy. Self-stigmatization is therefore the ultimate success for stigmatizers whose interest involves distorting their true motives and accepting the cultural assessment of the lower value of the stigmatized. The stigmatization processes help stigmatizers achieve their agendas through indirect, subtle, and taken-for-granted cultural circumstances (Link & Phelan 2014, 2).

Different social engagements–later in the book I present some examples like performances, exhibitions, and so on – are important mediators in these yet-to-be developed forms of sociotherapy, which demand that social members (not only survivors) change and promote the importance of change. However, most of these events do not adequately inform us of the power structure and symbolic power behind the (political) motives for maintaining the stigmatized status of war-rape survivors. One reason can apparently be found in the historically embedded structures of patriarchy, which can be simplified by looking at examples of survivors who have been abandoned or shamed within their own families for their "dirty" sexuality after being raped. The complex diversity of war experiences from a wider, top-down perspective occurs when we do not focus solely on the trauma of the rape survivor, but also take into consideration the fact that her husband, for instance, served as a camp guard or spent his time during the war in places that today are known for atrocities and violence against local inhabitants. Or another case, in which male family members of the female rape survivor, who stayed in the country during the war, were dragged into the complex war machinery. They are victims/survivors too – some as witnesses and, as hard as this is to acknowledge, as perpetrators, too. During my fieldwork between June and September of 2018,

I encountered three situations that further illustrate this. At this time, my focus was chiefly on women survivors and their traumatic stories. However, I struggled to continue the collaboration when I began collecting information – too much information – about their husbands and their activities during the war. These complexities have yet to be addressed, also in the context of stigmatization. When trying to understand survivors at the complex nexus of family relationships and intersectional/conflictual legacies from the war, one needs to assess the motives for stigmatization from the perspective of (symbolic) power and restorative/retributive justice. Nonetheless, the power structure that leads family members to abandon women survivors, the stigmatization and silence is not necessarily of a patriarchal nature. What if stigmatization is a mechanism that helps perpetrators obstruct justice and escape their crimes with impunity?

The responsibility for healing has now been imposed on survivors through the individualistic approach of psychotherapy and shared by members of the survivors' surrounding, which becomes a "silent majority"; the systematic and structural foundations that keep certain social members stigmatized and discriminated against is a natural extension of this psychosocial healing. While survivors invest time, energy, and sometimes money into their individual healing, the structure remains virtually unchanged. In one of the interviews that I conducted in June 2018 in Northeastern Bosnia, a survivor told me the following:

> As humans, we are emotional and rational beings. Psychotherapy is good for my emotions because when I go to the municipality or to any other institution, they give me papers and they do not need my emotions there. I need to fill in the data: where, what, when, who, how. Both my emotions and these data are needed to help us. But I have a feeling that I am cleaning these emotions, and someday I will feel I have left the past behind; I will not care about filling in the data, either. How then will criminals be prosecuted if I stop caring to report "the data"?
>
> (S62, Northeastern Bosnia 2018)

In another interview in Central Bosnia (2018), a survivor who had been taking antidepressants and painkillers for the past 15 years told me that she only needed to ensure that she could sleep at night:

> I feel so tired. I think I've given up. Look how fat I am? This is because I feel I can't fight this dysfunctional system, and my body is the reflection of it. I don't even go to the office[1] anymore because I've said it all and sharing it again and again is not benefiting me anymore. I think I've reached the final point; this is how I will remain for the rest of my life.
>
> (A60, Central Bosnia 2018)

When I asked the survivors during one of the workshops what their ideal "closure" to trauma would look like, one burst out, "To prosecute those who walk freely in these very streets every day" (A60, Central Bosnia 2018). Dealing with powerful political figures, particularly in today's corrupt, unstable, divided, and fragile postconflict Bosnia-Herzegovina is the most challenging part of healing; for some, it is even risky and dangerous. However, in the absence of stigma-power in anti-stigmatization projects, the focus is on stigma as a political weapon, which enables "the structures, mechanisms, and justifications of power to function" (Foucault 2008, 85) and will scarcely push the healing process forward.

To date, Goffman's stigma-concept has been taken up by social interactionalists, researching ways of communications and relationship between the individual (and self) and society (Goffman 1963; for a comprehensive review see: Crocker et al. 1998). Those theoretical paradigms have been perceived as "sociology from below," studying social interactions on a micro-level, and examining mostly everyday meaning production. Stigma-concept developed and used by social interactionists have been criticized for its over-emphasized notion on the power of individual agency in determining and/or changing the unjust, oppressive and suffering conditions they live in (Tyler and Slater 2018, 730–731). As a response, "political economy of stigmatization" (Parker and Aggleton 2003, 17) framed in stigma-power concept has introduced the structural inequalities, and larger political structures that consciously use the weapons of stigma to navigate desired behaviors, and control and retain existing hierarchies.

Macro-level structures and social relationships have come into the focus of resistance practices against stigmatization and have importantly turned the focus from individual (which is often oppressed and powerless in terms of economic and political means) to larger political bodies (Parker and Aggleton 2003; Pescosolido and Martin 2015). If applying stigma-power in the context of female war-rape survivors in Bosnia-Herzegovina, this turn can help one to reflect on individuals or/and collectives that deliberately employ stigmas to maintain the sociopolitical status quo of failed processes in retributive and restorative justice, particularly related to the questions of impunity and responsibility for the crimes. Social repercussions against survived women, justified through shaming and stigmatizing in their own communities, are working in favor of perpetrators: while stigma fosters the fear of ostracism, it prevents many survivors from reporting the crimes that consequently go unpunished.

In *The Stigma Complex*, published in the Annual Review of Sociology, Bernice Pescosolido and Jack Martin (2015, 101) emphasize that working with stigma means predominantly changing behaviors and beliefs rather than "changing the structures that shape social relationships." Drawing on Bourdieu's concept of symbolic power, stigma should be understood not as an omnipresent, apolitical, culturally transmitted social force but as "violence from above" (Wacquant 2008, 4), which operates as a "form of governance which legitimizes the reproduction and entrenchment of inequalities and injustices" (Tyler 2013, 212). Scholars who have been critical of Goffman's (1963) influential scholarship have dismissed the belief that individuals and social groups can be free of stigma if instructed how to better navigate stigma in social life or if the general public were educated about stigmatized conditions, factors, and actions (Tyler & Slater 2018, 729).

The impact of socially engaged initiatives is therefore crucial, not only in terms of retributive justice in the form of memory work, but in terms of paving a path toward justice in the prevention of sexual violence in current and future conflicts. Work with stigma-power emphasizes the development of systematic mechanisms that empower survivors to speak up by building alliances with citizens and important social (and religious) institutions. The inclusion of a criminal investigation component is essential, because it is one of the key promotors of impunity and stigma often reportedly used by individuals in power who are part of the criminal justice system. Without intending to consider the stigmatization of war-rape survivors in the multifaceted responses of the criminal justice system – at least in the long run – interventions in the "enclosure" phase will ultimately fail to break the stigma. Overestimating the role of individual social members in working with stigma while simultaneously downplaying the role of stigma-power reinforces rape myths and ignores the necessity for fundamental change in rape culture during times of both war and peace. Narrowly conceived interventions that include very specific and limited social circles and which fail to penetrate those social circles that foster both discursive and physical obstacles in the criminal prosecution of war rapes keep the issue of war-inflicted rape in the margins of political agendas.

While acknowledging the importance of random social members, it is important for "supporters" of integrating war-rape survivors into society to ease the pain of survivors' everyday lives. Stigma-power can only be broken, and healing can only progress if the individuals in question are no longer considered random citizens but instead constitute the structure(s) behind the act of stigmatization. What does the research on the perceptions of randomly selected war-rape survivors contribute to our knowledge of the mechanisms of stigmatization when we know little or nothing of their identities – their age, gender, social class, geographical location, and involvement/connection to war? I would argue that only by fully understanding how these individuals are embedded in the wider political structure can one understand the motives for the stigmatization of survivors.

As mentioned previously, the individual, let us say a mother, a survivor of war rape, can at the same time be a family member of two men who served in the army during the war and actively participated in combat. At some point during the war, one of these men was appointed as a guard in one of the detention camps, where he spent four months. While I had encountered this case, despite my best efforts, it was impossible to obtain more information about these two men's duties during the war and if/how they were involved in different war crimes, potentially including rapes. The healing of war-rape survivors cannot therefore be limited only to the survivor's psychological, intraprinciples of recovery; her experience must be incorporated into the wider aspect of postconflict recovery and reconciliation, taking into account that she still lives in an environment with others who have also survived, witnessed, and/or perpetrated the violence.

To be able to fully reintegrate war-rape survivors in the postwar society, I claim, one must look beyond the survivor-centered trauma healing and question the sociopolitical motivation behind the stigmatization in a such a long run after the war. In the following chapter I focus more concretely on the example of how the idea or survivor's silence is intentionally reproduced to sustain some of such motivations.

Narrated silences and the (ab)use of collective memory in sexual scripts

Whether one reads Slavenka Drakulić's classic novel *As If I Am Not There* (2001, 22), in which the protagonist – the victim of war-related rape – keeps "swallowing not only / ... / words, but even / ... / thoughts," or watches the dramatization of the same work by Juanita Wilson (2009), the portrayal of women raped during the war in Bosnia in the 1990s communicates the same message: the omnipresence of *silence* is embodied in the very way the characters exist. They "walk with hunched shoulders, their eyes lowered, their bodies pressed together, and quiet, making themselves smaller than they are" (Drakulić 2001, 45). In a 2006 film by Jasmila Žbanić, released in the United Kingdom as *Esma's Secret: Grbavica*, the main protagonist, Esma, portrays this nexus of silence, shame, and secrets as the representative of "raped Bosnia." Esma is mostly a quiet, passive woman, and her ongoing fear – which we can see in her wide open but still insecure eyes – is continuously narrated through her perpetual silence: from the very beginning, when her eyes open abruptly to seek empathy with the spectator, to "dropping her head and keeping silent" (Vojnović 2006).

The ubiquity of the silence that surrounds the crime of war rape and its aftermath among survivors is visible not only in narratives of eternal victimhood and innocence but also in the recurring titles of works on rape: *Breaking the Wall of Silence* (1996), *The Silent Scream* (2014), and *Sound of Silence* (2014), to name just a few. Those titles play with the semantic contradiction of silence and scream; moreover, breaking, and screaming all signify acts of resistance, the active against the passive, and therefore exert a control which suggests that silence is a deliberate choice of the survivors. The 2014 documentary movie title *The Silent Scream* (*Nečujni krik*), produced by Balkan Investigative Reporting Group (BIRN), for instance, communicates two extreme psychological anxieties that survivors usually experience: on the one hand, the burden of embodied trauma and overwhelming urges *to scream out*, and, on the other hand, the social pressure to remain silent and its repercussions in the process of stigmatization and exclusion (see also Culbertson 1995).

Delić and Avdibegović (2016) report that survivors of rapes committed during the war in Bosnia in the 1990s often expressed the fear that their stories would not be heard or that people would simply not be able to understand what had happened to them. Those survivors who contributed their testimonies mentioned an inability to talk with their spouses and even talked of being abandoned after they spoke out. They generally felt that they could not trust others, and silence appeared to be the best response for their self-recovery, especially while trying to leave the past behind and move on with their lives. Given such consequences, the executive producer of *The Silent Scream*, Mirna Buljugić, sees the significance of the movie as addressing the culture of silence perpetuated by communities and social circles surrounding the survivors. In the words of Erna Mackic, editor at the BIRN Bosnia-Herzegovina office, "society is not ready to hear them, listen, or help" (Justice Report 2014). A journalist who reported on the movie added: "The core of this trepidation is due to the incident itself; nobody really feels at ease when talking about surviving a rape. But the silence is reinforced by aspects of Bosnian society, a predominantly traditional society with a male power monopoly" (Ferizaj 2015).

While unease when listening to rape stories remains, I believe that the processes involved in "speaking the silence" have changed enormously; so too have the uses of the "silence" paradigm in today's processes of reconciliation and social recovery. Before introducing the ways in which these silences are intentionally narrated today, I would like to first take a detour into a more general understanding of how silence among survivors is a constantly changing process and how the silence related to sexual violence differs from the dynamics of silences that have been recorded by survivors of other (collective) crimes.

Many studies have repeatedly confirmed that trauma survivors keep the details of their painful past experiences secret (Danieli 1998; Kidron 2009). As George Simmel argued in his classic essay "The Secret and Secret Society," a sense of community is built from a consciously desired concealment that enables group cohesion by restricting the distribution of social knowledge. With the help of such concealment, the community controls the system of power and directs moral conduct. In the context of Holocaust survivors, several authors have defined this silence in terms of *unspeakability* (Caruth 1995; Kidron 2009), or the inability to discursively frame the nature of a horrific experience. Caruth (1995) and other scholars asserted that trauma is fundamentally incomprehensible, unreadable, and inaccessible, and other authors have maintained the same stance on silence as "signifying the ineffability of the disaster" (Blanchot 1986) and the limits of ethically narrating the atrocities of war and genocide (see Adorno 1949; White 1992; La Capra 1994). Bar-On (1996) describes silence as a result of the "primary pain of the trauma and the victims' consequent difficulty in putting this pain into words" (Bar-On 1996, 99), which eventually makes this pain "indescribable." According to Bar-On, the victims' pain manifests itself in the social responses of certain bystanders which transform perpetrators' atrocities into silenced facts.

Hence, the silence of survivors is not solely the consequence of indescribable psychological and physiological pain, but rather the combination of individual pain and the social representation that dehumanizes and humiliates victims as human beings (Anderson & Doherty 2008; Ullman 2010). The nonverbalized expression of the unspeakable nature of traumatic experience is beyond the narrative. Devastating traumatic events are believed to create ruptures in the linear flow of experience – a disruption that resists any attempts at verbal representation (Caruth 1995). Silence among survivors is often understood to signify psychological and political repression. Because it deviates from the Eurocentric psychosocial norm of voice, the absence of voice, according to Kidron (2009, 6), signals "psychopathologized processes of avoidance and repression, socially suspect processes of personal secrecy, or collective processes of political subjugation." Introducing "narrated silences" overshadows the attempt to understanding why the pain of survivors is "indescribable." Consequently, it turns our focus toward the processes in the surrounding environment that use this "inability" to describe to transform the silences into intentionally "undiscussable" social realities.

Silence in the context of sexual abuse is never only an absence of communication, of speaking openly of the atrocities, or an inability to verbalize the abuse – it becomes a part of depriving the body of the survivor of her mind and ego. The complexity of silence among rape survivors is exacerbated by the fact that sexuality is, with rare exceptions across time and cultures, suppressed and "silenced." Sexual taboos, social stigmas, and different fears are also communicated through silence in terms of the broader, toxic social context, in which speaking out is not simply a matter of reporting a crime, but more a question of honour and shame (see Skjelsabek 2011). Most aspects of human sexuality are articulated in the forms of "taboos against looking, listening, as well as speaking" (Zerubavel 2010, 34). Silence is used as a means to defend their honour, which is their sexuality, as a morally and physically pure female essence. To respond with silence is to accept that moral misconduct here is not *the rape*, but *being raped*. In this context, the women raped and subjected to silence become manifestations of a kind of social punishment. Silence about war rapes, therefore, helps members of society and social groups to position themselves in response to the judgments of others.

While silence sometimes appears as the consequence of a secret – part of a painful past that cannot be communicated aloud – survivors report that they also remain silent because of the desire to forget past traumas in order to construct new, trauma-free, postwar identities. In this way, silence becomes a vehicle of *comfortable discomfort*; when many have yet to work through the overwhelming legacy of the past, silence offers at least a certain predictability. The survivor uses silence to deny and ignore the past so that she might move on with her life (and her family) constructively, without being preoccupied with danger. It is therefore problematic to perceive silence, or the inability to speak out, only in negative terms. Deciding to leave the past behind – attempting to bury it in one's own memory – might backfire; but it might also help the survivor to recover. One of the survivor's tells me:

> I have been silent for almost 12 years. Then I was invited by /.../ and for the first time I told what happened to me. It was very big. I cried and cried. Before I was just living in fear of being discovered, but after I told /.../ I just cried. I only told this once. Now I still come here /to the association/ and other women always speak again and again, but I just listen. I am now a grandmother, I see my grandson, and this is what I care about. I also wish others would stop saying again and again what has happened, we've already heard! But who knows, maybe they need this as I need them to stop talking about this.
>
> (R, Central Bosnia 2018)

In continuing the conversation, I learned that sharing her story was important for her; however, it was also clear that not repeating the testimony was important in her approach to recovery. When we speak about the silences, we assume that silence is a simple, fixed, finished, and stable state from which survivors can cope with their traumas, and that this is a unique form of silence that can be recognized among traumatized individuals. In doing so, we ignore the dynamics within which individuals can engage with the silences over time, as well as the social circles within which survivors can share their story. Later in the book I give the example where one survivor feels completely comfortable sharing her story with children in a region other than her own but would never talk about her experience at the school close to her home, for example. To understand the complexities involved in silence and in speaking out, I suggest looking at the relationship between the survivors and the silence in four levels (Figure 3.1):

DISENGAGED
TRAUMATIC EVENT → NOT LISTENING NOR SHARING & MOVING AWAY

PASSIVE TO ACTIVE
TRAUMATIC EVENT → LISTENING TO OTHER WITHOUT EVER SHARING OR ENGAGING

ACTIVE TO PASSIVE
TRAUMATIC EVENT → SPEAKING OUT → LISTENING TO THE OTHERS WITHOUT FURTHER ENGAGEMENTS

ENGAGED
TRAUMATIC EVENT → SPEAKING OUT → LISTENING TO THE OTHERS → SPEAKING OUT → ∞

Figure 3.1 Levels of survivor's engagement.

Based on the estimated number of rapes (between 20,000 and 50,000) and the number of registered survivors (or those who spoke about this), one can assume that the largest number of survivors decided to remain silent. Little is known about the recovery and struggles of those individuals. In addition, with the pressures involved in speaking out, little focus was given to the methodologies employed to approach or discuss those silences. Might these survival strategies actually work better for those who remain silent, or should we assume that the large proportion of survivors suffers in isolated silence? When someone decides to remain silent with the goal of moving away from the trauma of the past, and where this silence is perceived as resilience in the same way as speaking out and advocating, we need to understand if those silences are effective in preventing the transmission of trauma. Based on past knowledge, we came to agree that speaking out and other active approaches to dealing with trauma help both psychological and social recovery.

However, my encounters with both mothers and children have raised plenty of doubt and hesitancy about what has appeared to be a dogmatic approach to dealing with silence and trauma. Although the decision to remain silent is somehow accepted as the legitimate right of survivors (in trying to understand

their difficulties, lack of support, strengths, and resources), the powerful exposure of those who in fact did speak out, and were widely applauded as *heroines*,
establishes certain hierarchical positions and occasional bitterness as to why some
put more effort into finding solutions while others reap the benefits. As we have
no strong and reliable ethnographic evidence – and no method to decode silences
and silent individuals but only assumptions and conclusions based on the words
of those who speak – we can understand the *disengaged* position of those survivors. However, in the existing hierarchical order of silence versus speech, "disengaged" cannot be used without risking a negative connotation. I suggest that
we reclaim this position, understanding disengagement as a process of "moving
away" – if not "moving forward" – and embracing the disengaged position with a
commitment to further developing methodological approaches and epistemological understanding.

Along the way, I have met survivors who have been regularly present, attending activities organized in the framework of their associations or just sympathiz-
ing, but who have never really shared their own stories; perhaps they shared some
pieces of it, or they seconded the thoughts of others who spoke out. However,
they listened. This brings us back to what I mentioned above, that our understanding of silence is still too often limited to the absence of speech; yet the
bodily presence of survivors, the fact that they respond with listening, perhaps
commenting, giving feedback, is all part of *speaking out*. Now, how do we deal
with such "silence"? In a case such as this, is it important to push forward and
to put her own story into words? Based on observations in similar contexts, I
would claim that *active listening* has been as powerful as speaking out for many
survivors, as well as being less traumatizing. In addition, survivors who participate only as active listeners offer important but unacknowledged support to
those who speak. Creating circles of trust and physical presence is essential to
empower those who perform and advocate in public. Again, while speaking has
a hierarchical lead and is perceived as active (as opposed to "passive" silence),
listening and physical presence and support without speaking are overlooked as
valuable means of support.

Another dynamic involves a survivor deciding to share her story, after which
she does not participate in terms of speaking but remains active as a listener or
"silent" supporter. In one of the workshops in 2018, I have asked survivors about
the repetitive cycle of sharing testimonies, and most expressed the feeling that
telling a story again and again is rather burdensome, as opposed to being cathartic
or therapeutic. One survivor explained that repeating her story to different professionals and through different media is important to reach those responsible and to
trigger a reaction; however, she clearly expressed her disappointment that, having
shared her testimony numerous times in numerous places to numerous professionals, there were few actual long-term benefits and constructive outcomes of
this process.

The paradoxical fact is that the knowledge that we have today concerning silence
is, in the end, mostly built on the words of those who have spoken; everything
else – that is, the silence itself – is based on assumptions and conclusions drawn

from the available evidence, which consists mostly of speech and writing. Our existing knowledge and the narrative about silenced survivors is based on a very particular analysis of the dynamics – an analysis that is constructed on the basis of observations that we are capable of comprehending. This also explains why today – despite a rich collection of testimonies from those who have spoken out – we continue to talk about "silenced survivors." Furthermore, with the increased participation of survivors in public life, the recognition and approval of narratives of silence and silent survivors has become stronger over the past 25 years. It has become an inevitable part of survivors' identities almost without exception. While the numbers of survivors who expose themselves publicly *by speaking out* has increased, different stakeholders – including academics and journalists – are still responsible for the continued reproduction of the "silent survivor" narrative. Although survivors have different backgrounds and have had different experiences of rape and recovery in the aftermath of the war, we hear little about any narrative other than the narrative of silence (see also Mookherjee 2006).

Reflecting back on the postwar recovery and reintegration of survivors, where little or nothing is known and promised to survivors should they decide to break their silence, and where life has not changed dramatically for the better for those who have decided to speak out, what is the motivation today for those who remain silent? Why – if not for matters of personal recovery – would one decide to do the work that is in fact the work of each of us who constitute the surrounding society? Why do we not address collected testimonies instead of pushing the silent ones to speak out? How many testimonies would be enough to successfully achieve the changes that survivors demand in the process of transitional and restorative justice?

Acknowledging the dynamics of silence is important; first, it removes the burden on survivors to repeat their stories over and over again, enabling them to move on and to live beyond this story. Second, it would prevent revictimization and also acknowledge the contributions of those who remain silent but offer support in other ways (physical presence, active listening, etc.). Third, it would encourage us, as professionals in the field, to further develop methodologies and applicative, empirical work with those who remain silent. Fourth, and most importantly for the scope of this book, understanding that the same survivors speak out in circles of others survivors remain silent in their families would guide us in wrestling with the questions of trauma transmission that occur between mothers and their offspring.

There is another dynamic that I did not add to the above table, and I omitted it for the reason that it includes main actors who are not survivors. Whereas Helsinki Watch (1993) and Amnesty International (1993) published reports of rapes that they had gathered while the war was ongoing, the above mentioned cross-sectional study by Delić and Avdibegović (2016) shows that the average period of silence for most survivors is approximately ten years. This lapse not only explains the flood of literature on different aspects of the phenomenon of war rape in Bosnia-Herzegovina from around the same time, but also shows who was in charge to deal with the silence – trying to describe it and frame it theoretically; and "break" it within the practices of psychosocial support and activism. Even as survivors long resisted speaking out, academics and journalists were committed to breaking the silence and even to working against the "conspiracy of silence' (Danieli 1998; Zerubavel 2010). We can read these attempts as Kidron (2009, 8) described them: "moral and political mission[s]" in which the anthropologist-turned-activist liberates trauma victims from the "shadows of silence' (Waterston & Rylko-Bauer 2006). A popular culture production shows that the diversity of applied formats did not contribute to the questioning and challenging of those silences, but rather the opposite: appropriations of survivors' testimonies often serve to reinforce existing representations.

In the two decades since the Dayton Peace Agreement of 1995, the "silenced survivor" paradigm has become a "debased currency" and "a modish idea" (Leys 2000, 304) within interested academic circles and among the broader public. I claim that today, more than ever, the conversation about silence, like silence itself, has been subject to a "complex of negotiations about what is acceptable and what is to be silenced, what can and cannot be said, in the disjunctions between private narratives and public discourses" (Jelin 2003, 16). However, I believe that the reader will agree with me that, following the release of Angelina Jolie's (in)famous 2011 feature movie *In the Land of Blood and Honey* – in which rapes and raped women are the protagonists – the history of war rape in Bosnia-Herzegovina today is "generally known but cannot be spoken" (Taussig 1999, 51). The status of war rapes today is beyond the "silent witnessing" in which the conspirator is aware of his crimes but is unwilling to publicly acknowledge them (Cohen 2001, 75). Rather, the paradigm of survivor silence is intentionally being recreated, reproduced, and applied to the needs of the current sociopolitical context. On several occasions, I have witnessed individuals using the contradictory syntax, *talking-about-silence*. But isn't talking about the silence that surrounds rapes already talking and therefore breaking the silence? Being troubled by this complex dynamic, I wrote in my diary:

> I am confused about the attachment that survivors have to the idea of silence. It is striking for me to spend time with survivors listening how no one wants to listen to them, how they are being shut down and silenced, and then scrolling through the Facebook page of their organization and following all the posts that are obviously not only 'breaking the silence' but sharing knowledge on matters related to the legal and psychological dimensions of the active survivors behind the posts. I keep wondering why there is this attachment, why they keep using the "silence" when it is obvious to me that, in these times of Facebook and other social media, they have familiarized themselves with the technology and are very courageously using the power of those platforms. More and more, it seems to me that there are, as elsewhere, two separate spaces – one being the traditional, "real" world where I assume the silence still pertains. Somehow, I came to understand that it is challenging for them to speak openly and as much as they would want with their beloved,

their family members, or maybe the community. And when they post on Facebook about being silent, perhaps they are referring to the traditional, physical spaces where they live. But then I wonder where and how we place the silence and, moreover, what it is that women need and find more important, both in terms of their own healing and social reintegration: to be loud and vocal on seemingly "non-personal" but powerful platforms such as Facebook, where they can remain "victims" or "survivors" as a collective, or to "break through" in their own very local environment, where they are no longer a part of the collective but a member of the community, with a name, a face, and a very singular and very personal story.

(2019)

I call this attachment, where silence is represented as a supposedly unique survivors' response to rape, but which has in fact *a strong political and ideological motif, narrated silence*. Narrated silence(s) contribute to strengthening the existing, oppressive, heterosexual scripts in which the sexual autonomy of women is neglected. The silence surrounding war rapes in Bosnia-Herzegovina is neither random nor spontaneous; it is systematically reproduced to maintain existing sociopolitical orders that are counterproductive on both individual and collective levels. Individually, the narrated silence disables survivors, preventing them from recovering and moving on with their lives; collectively, it prevents justice for targeted social groups and simultaneously threatens to transmit the idea of acceptable, non-punished (unprosecuted), violent, and nonconsensual heterosexuality (see, for instance, Cliff 1978; Vincent & Durham 2014; Delić & Avdibegović 2016). In reducing survivors to speechless and voiceless spectacles of victimization, the use of narrated silence contributes significantly to problematic identities for survivors and to relationship dynamics that often normalize gender-based violence, abuse, or nonconsensual intercourse as part of the culturally accepted sexual culture.

At the same time, speaking out is also a part of the narrated silences, as it "warns" survivors that breaking the silence might risk destabilization of the social habitus and intimate relationships. The decision to remain silent is believed to protect the dignity and respect of survivors in their communities: speaking up eventually decreases their individual trauma but increases the risk of being social rejected and shunned by families and friends. In addition to social stigma, past studies reveal that survivors' stories have been regularly silenced by postconflict (nationalistic) projects and the imposed cultural imperative of the "unspeakability" of wartime rapes (see Agathangelou 2000; Hayden 2000; Ruff-O'Herne 2008). This contextual yet omnipresent pressure offers optimal conditions for the nurturing of rape culture among postwar generations. In the context of war-rape survivors and the public recognition of rape as a crime, therefore, the narrated silence operates not only in private, but also in a political space where information is manipulated. The negotiation of silence and recognition participates discursively and empirically in constructing societies, social order, and new hierarchies in the aftermath of war.

Evidence of silence among survivors has always been amplified through diverse genres, allowing the silence paradigm to become publicly recognized, accepted and, consequently, unquestioned. Survivors' fears that their testimonies will not be believed or will be appropriated, and that they will therefore be revictimized (Henry 2010) all add to the vicious, unbreakable cycle of silence that follows rape. Theoretical and empirical endorsement of the *narrated silence* is rather problematic; when we frame historical accounts of rapes within broader, semifictional narratives, we transmit ideological and metaphorical acknowledgment of certain cultural patterns, particularly those controlling female sexuality and reinforcing traditional gender roles. While the number of survivors sharing their testimonies has been increasing in recent years, the narrative of silence has been "self-reinforcing" (Bird 1996, 51). The longer we remain silent, the more silence we need to cover the previous silences. In other words, "silence becomes more prohibitive the longer it lasts" (Bird 1996, 51). In this way, silence becomes an essential part of the collective memory of survivors, creating "a complex and rich social space that can operate as a vehicle of either memory or of forgetting and thus can be used by various groups for different ends" (Vinitzky-Seroussi & Teeger 2010, 1104). In Durkheimian terms, collective memory is the center of the means of social production (for more, see Eyerman 2004) – silence, as a part of that memory, constitutes a foundation for different cultural scripts (Plummer 1995).

Accepting silence as it is represented and reproduced through new narratives also means accepting the culture of rape. The silences that surround rape are the prolonged silences surrounding sexuality in general. Sexuality has been silenced continuously, and just as practices, rituals, and beliefs both normative and alternative have coexisted empirically, so too did the agreement about sexuality as a matter that is private, hidden, and enigmatic. While debate about sexuality was (and still is) socially controlled, normalized sexuality essentially became its own manifestation of silence. Narrated silences of war-rape survivors have been approached with medicalized and individualized treatments for a long time, normalizing – if not symbolically justifying – the isolation of survivors. These silences seldom point to other actors – not only perpetrators, but allies, family members, and society in general. Although speaking out is essential so that the crimes are not forgotten, today's acknowledgment and knowledge of rape demonstrate what Susan Sontag (2003) calls not remembering, but stipulating: that this is important, that this is the story of how it happened, with pictures that lock the story in our minds. Ideologies create substantiating archives of images, representative images, which encapsulate common ideas of significance and trigger predictable thoughts and feelings (Sontag 2003, 86).

Silence, framed in memory, becomes a "collective instruction" (Sontag, ibid.) through which the past continues and shapes the present on three levels (after Schudson 1997): (a) *personally*, through how it is transmitted in individual lives; (b) *socially*, as manifested in social institutions and laws; and (c) *culturally*, mainly through language and symbolic systems. The narrated collective memory of survivors' sexuality, when limited to abuse and silence, therefore supports

patriarchal, oppressive norms, cultural perspectives, understandings of relationships, gender-related paradigms, values, and beliefs. The experience of war rapes
only confirms the normativity of violent sexuality and women's acceptance of that
norm. The ways in which a culture defines and understands "appropriate" sexual
practices and gender roles mediate the silence and shame of sexual victimization rather than criminal sexual perpetuation. In societies such as that of Bosnia-
Herzegovina, women's chastity, moral laws concerning what is "good and bad,"
sexist imagery, and the assumed superiority of men and male heterosexuality, as
well as the cultural legacy of taboos, stigmas, and silence from prewar times, all
(in)directly impact the perceptions and representations of war-rape survivors.

When the occurrence of war rapes communicated through narrated silences
constitutes such an important part of collective memory, it becomes part of our
sexual scripts (Plummer 1995). As with any other socialization process, the narrated silences of war rapes are operated by three important agents. First are (a) *the
producers*, who turned themselves into social, sexual objects. They display their
sexual lives and provide stories to spectators and audiences. Both language and
the silence of trauma provide societies with their ideas about sexuality and sexual
violence. Survivors' narratives play crucial roles here in exposing oppression,
violence, and trauma; giving voice to "silent histories" raises awareness and public recognition of gender-based violence and "alters history's narrative" (Hesford
1999, 195). Every one of us who reproduces these narrated silences collaborates
in this process. We create the image of what happens/what should happen with
survivors after rape: her response, her personal efforts in recovery, her struggles.
Moreover, and this is disturbing, as producers we navigate our response as social
actors, passive or active, witnesses or allies.

Those targeted by the stories might become either (b) *coaxers* or (c) *consumers*.
Coaxers are listeners and questioners; the coaxer, for instance, is the researcher
who brings problematic narratives of silence and shame to the public and attempts
to shatter the stigma of sexually abused women. Consumers consume stories
as narrated, or interpret them through their accepted social conceptualizations
(Plummer 1995, 106–107). The consumer does not take into consideration the
contextual meaning of the consumed material and its (harmful) long-term impacts.
A coaxer, on the other hand, is an agent who shifts the focus from the survivors
to the matter of assigning responsibility from the surrounding context. Coaxers
might contribute to the shifting narratives and, over longer periods, shifting social
patterns; however, it seems that society hungers only for consumption. For it is
not at all surprising to me that, despite new knowledge and general changes in
social structures and organizations over the last 25 years, the same narratives are
repeated over and over again. The meanings of the stories depend, of course, not
only on the actors, but on changes in the realms of context and associated social
worlds (Plummer 1995, 106).

Sexual scripts are a "set of behaviours, beliefs, and the meanings attached to
them [which] are constructed by individuals and social groups" and can change
over time and across national boundaries (Lewis 2006, 254). The rape, the violence, the pleasure, the visibility, and the denial of (female) sexuality are defined

by these scripts, but as Lewis (2006, 256) argues, they are "not simply down-loaded verbatim into individuals. They select the cultural scenarios that are most consistent with their own ideas of and experiences with sexuality and incorporate them into their own menu of sexual acts." However, narrated silences can impose dangerous intrapsychic scripts, in which sexual meanings and desires serve as a guide for sexual conduct, not only in the present but also in our understanding of the past and in our future actions (Laumann & Gagnon 1995; Whittier & Simon 2001). Intrapsychic scripts include fantasies, memories, and mental rehearsals, and it is within these intrapsychic scripts that individuals work out the difficulties involved in enacting interpersonal scripts within the general context of cultural scenarios (Simon & Gagnon 1986).

Some scholars would oppose this thesis by claiming that the narrated silence is indeed the portrayal of the actual silence and is primarily used in families as a protective mechanism (Bar-On 1996; Wiseman & Barber 2008). Survivors who want to forget the past and adjust to new, postconflict lives continue to believe that withholding information about the horrors they experienced is compulsory for their children's unaffected development. Past studies have shown that this belief is a misconception: children who were "protected" from the traumatic stories of their parents and grandparents were sometimes affected by ill health, social dysfunction, community violence, and other outcomes (for more, see Milroy 2005). The nonverbal transmission of ideas, the silent presence of the individual's violent experience in the past, is an important form of communication that reproduces existing patterns of rape culture and oppressive sexual scripts. According to Waynryb (2001), survivor–descendant interactions entail transmitting shared ideas or meanings as a system of signs.

Silence, denial, and shame – all (un)discursive practices that surround the legacy of rape – help to maintain a conception of sexual violence in which women are viewed as "inherently rapable" (Smith 2005, 3). Recent history, rape stories both told and untold, and the ethnic stereotypes that remain embedded in every piece of cultural identity render survivors and their families more vulnerable to sexual stigmatization; more disturbingly, the men and boys on the other side are no less stigmatized: a male becomes subjected to positioning as a rapist and a perpetrator. Transmitted trauma thus manifests itself through narrated silences and translates into rape myths (Burt 1980) – prejudicial, stereotyped ideas, perceptions, and beliefs about rape, rape victims, and rape perpetrators.

How then, if we keep reproducing narratives that promote narrated silences, are we to include the history and legacy of sexual violence and their traumatic consequences into peace education? Some scholars (see Blanco & Rosa 1997; Egan 1997) have proposed that the teaching of historical events should promote critical and reflexive approaches, whereby the past is understood not as a series of definite events but as a constructed and sometimes unfaithful representation of shifting social realities. This certainly applies to the sociology of sexuality, wherein the latter is no longer presented as a naturalized, normalized, and unchanging biological instinct but as shaped by learning and socialization processes. "Breaking the silence" – that is, teaching about war rape in conflicts – is, therefore, not about teaching certain historical events; this instruction should promote the critical positioning of histories of sexuality. What we might learn from this historical experience is that silence provides a narrative frame for rape stories to be told out loud and, at the same time, for survivors to stay protected.

Accepting the silence of raped women as the "most dignified position" means accepting a whole set of established sexual identities, power balances, and relationships. Narrated silences therefore send problematic messages to future generations of girls and boys. For girls, the narrated silence is a sexual script of acceptance of abusive sexuality; at the same time, this narrative teaches them how to become "real" victims (by not speaking up). On the other hand, the very same silence assures boys that their crimes will not be made public and/or punished; hence, rape is legitimized and tolerated. When narrated silences are thus translated into accepted and normalized cultural scenarios, we are no longer dealing with the past of survivors; rather, this past begins to haunt succeeding generations and indirectly affects their social realities. Teaching about the war rapes that happened two decades ago is no longer in the domain of historical writing, but has become an important learning moment in social and political education. In this vein, understanding silence as it relates to sexual crimes – its construction, function, and use – is as much a constitutive part of peacebuilding activities as any other silence.

The narrated silence might operate as the crucial and sometimes sole source of information for youngsters accessing the stories of their parents. As such, the narrated silences intervene powerfully in the spheres of nonformal education and socialization; they not only inform the past but, more importantly, they suggest how to incorporate the lessons and experiences of the past into existing sets of values, viewpoints, and cultural (sexual) scripts. For this reason, any re-creation and/or reproduction of narratives that can communicate the normalization of harmful social relations, dynamics, or processes holds us as creators responsible to fortify the efforts of critical mediation and the reading of constructed social realities. It is not too extreme to say that silence – such as an *absence* of women's testimonies or an absence of evidence – does not exist. If hundreds of recorded and archived testimonies still count as *silence*, then we should be directed toward employing another, related term – denial. To successfully pursue denial on the side of all interested parties, silence will always be a convenient controlling mechanism with which to operate.

The efforts of various individuals and groups have brought to light enough evidence for us to hear what has happened. A rich knowledge of war-rape crimes (not only in Bosnia, but worldwide) is now accessible nationally and internationally; the voices of women have certainly been present in very different arenas, from courts and community hubs to traditional and social media. Instead of empowering those voices and trying to hear them, we lean on those who, for various reasons, have decided to remain silent. Hence, not silences but *narrated* silences are one of the greatest discursive and empirical anomalies in the epistemological legacy of war rapes and survivors, as narratives of "unspeakability" and silence have been made on the basis of the testimonies of those who actually spoke out.

Does the prevailing myth of silence mean that the silence will finally be broken only when all 50,000 or so victims decide to speak out? Are those the only circumstances in which we, as a society, will be able to move on and acknowledge the urgent need to reformulate the entire idea of how we narrate rape in general?

Knowing that the exact number of violated women has never been confirmed and is regularly disputed, there will then always be reason for us to say, "Rape survivors remain silent." In the 1970s, when Holocaust studies started to discover the impact of silence on the transmission of trauma, every survivor's testimony counted: the modes of recording and distributing the awareness of the past crimes were limited, both in terms of reaching the audience and impacting the general society. Today, in an era of powerful audio-visual communications, rapid information sharing, greater awareness of the importance of speaking up, reporting, and sharing, the paradigm of survivors' silences might even appear artificial. For many, as the narrative continues to present women survivors as powerless, shut down, and voiceless, narrated silences have become ideological vehicles for the preservation of – and advocacy for – heteronormative values. Returning to the image of the silent victim rather than the vocal survivor confirms the broader sociopolitical demand for the preservation and support of these categories and identities. Although different actors have aimed to bring the topic of war-rape survivors to the fore – and have, to some extent, succeeded – the reoccurring presence of the narrated silence reaffirms and empowers the many social myths it was supposed to combat. If the silence does indeed exist as narrated, then isn't the knowledge we have about survivors a mere interpretation of those who do have the voice and ability to speak about those crimes?

In a postconflict Bosnia-Herzegovina that remains a vulnerable and psychologically unrecovered territory, I believe that narrated silence is thoughtfully planned and institutionally welcomed. Although war and conflict might sometimes offer a space for social change and the restructuring of sociopolitical systems, narrated silences keep alive the harmful prewar environment for women – and at the end for everyone – promoting essentialist understandings of sexualities and gender roles. Only by resisting the reproduction of this narrative can we resist, also, the perpetrators' efforts to remain protected and unpunished. On this note, I suggest two directions for further thinking and writing about war-rape survivors and the legacy of war rape in postconflict contexts. The first is to shift the narrative focus away from individualized and medicalized social perceptions of survivors. This also means a decentralization in terms of the holistic and contextual conceptualization of war rape. There is plenty of silence on the perpetrators' side; we miss, almost completely, this side of the story. But beyond these polarized war roles, victim and perpetrator, much can be done by the actors in between: witnesses, observers, analysts, and allies. We need to start recognizing that reproduced narratives – like narrated silences – can transmit toxic messages and work toward transforming them into constructive social instructions.

For this, I proposed earlier the importance of understanding the evolution, nuanced dynamics, normalization, and institutionalization of the silences surrounding the sexuality of raped individuals. This understanding might, furthermore, help us to pay more attention to silence as a socially imposed and desired position, rather than a response to the unbearable trauma that rape causes to individuals. This would furthermore bring us to the understanding that it is not the responsibility of survivors to break the silence, but the responsibility of the surrounding society to intervene in the genres and narratives that reproduce the paradigm of silence – a silence that disables survivors, impeding their healing and reintegration into society.

Note

1 The organization's office and place where women meet on a weekly basis.

Bibliography

Adorno, T. 1949. *Gesellschaftstheorie und Kulturkritik*. Frankfurt am Mein: Suhrkamp.

Agathangelou, A. M. 2000. "Nationalist narratives and (dis)appearing women: State sanctioned sexual violence." *Canadian Woman Studies* 19 (4): 12–21.

Akman, K. B. 2015. "Sociotherapy as a contemporary alternative." *Bangladesh E-Journal of Sociology* 12 (1): 9–16.

Allen, B. 1996. *Rape warfare: The hidden genocide in Bosnia-Herzegovina and Croatia*. Minneapolis: University of Minnesota Press.

Amnesty International. 1993. *Bosnia-Herzegovina: Rape and sexual abuse by armed forces*. London: International Secretariat.

Anderson, I. and Doherty, K. 2008. *Accounting for rape*. London: Routledge.

Bar-On, D. 1996. *The indescribable and the undiscussable: Reconstructing human discourse after trauma*. Budapest: Central European University.

Barry, K. 1979. *Female sexual slavery*. Englewood Cliffs, NJ: Prentice-Hall.

Berry, M. E. 2017. "Barriers to women's progress after atrocity: Evidence from Rwanda and Bosnia-Herzegovina." *Gender and Society* 31 (6): 830–853.

Bird, F. B. 1996. *The muted conscience: Moral silence and the practice of ethics in business*. Westport, CT: Quorum Books.

BIRN Justice Report. 2014. "Documentary 'Silent Scream' shown in Sarajevo." Available at http://www.balka ninsi ght.com/en/artic le/birn-docum entar y-silen t-screa m-premi ers-in-saraj evo (accessed 18 November 2019).

Blanchot, M. 1986. *The writing of the disaster*. London: University of Nebraska Press.

Blanco, F. and Rosa, A. 1997. "Dilthey's dream: Teaching history to understand the future." *International Journal of Educational Research* 27 (3): 189–200.

Burt, M. R. 1980. "Cultural myths and supports for rape." *Journal of Personality and Social Psychology* 38 (2): 217–230.

Caruth, C. 1995. "Recapturing the past: Introduction." In C. Caruth (Ed.), *Trauma: Explorations in memory* (151–157). Baltimore: Johns Hopkins University Press.

Clark, N. J. 2016. "Working with survivors of war rape and sexual violence fieldwork reflections from Bosnia-Hercegovina." *Qualitative Research* 17 (4): 424–439.

Cliff, M. 1978. "Notes on speechlessness." *Sinister Wisdom* 5 (Winter 1978): 5–9.

Cohen, S. 2001. *States of denial. Knowing about atrocities and suffering*. Cambridge: Cambridge University Press.

Crocker, J., Major, B., and Steele, C. 1998. "Social stigma." In S. Fiske, D. Gilbert and G. Lindzey (Eds.), *Handbook of Social Psychology* (504–553). Boston, MA: McGraw-Hill.

Culbertson, R. 1995. "Embodied memory, transcendence, and telling: Recounting trauma, Re-Establishing the Self." *New Literary History* 26 (1): 169–195.

Danieli, Y. 1998. "Introduction: History and conceptual foundations." In Y. Danieli (Ed.), *International handbook of multigenerational legacies of trauma* (1–17). New York: Plenum.

Davies, W. 2017. "On mental health, the royal family is doing more than our government." Available at https://www.theguardian.com/commentisfree/2017/ apr/20/m (accessed 8 July 2019).

Delić, A. and Avdibegović, E. 2016. "Shame and silence in the aftermath of war rape in Bosnia and Herzegovina: 22 years later." Available at https://www.researchgate.net/p ublication/293815848_Shameand_Silence_in_the_aftermath_of_War_Rape_in_Bosni a_and_Herzegovina_22_years later (accessed 5 November 2019).

Drakulić, S. 2001. *As if I am not there*. London: Hachette Digital.

Edelson, M. 1970. *Sociotherapy and psychotherapy*. Chicago: University of Chicago Press.

Egan, K. 1997. *The educated mind: How cognitive tools shape our understanding*. Chicago: University of Chicago Press.

Eyerman, R. 2004. "The past in the present culture and the transmission of memory." *Acta Sociologica* 47 (2): 159–169.

Felman, S. and Laub, D. 1991. *Testimony: Crises of witnessing in literature, psychoanalysis and history*. New York: Routledge.

Ferizaj, A. 2015. "Insight into Bosnia-and-Herzegovina's male and female survivors of wartime rape." Available at https://www.opendemocracy.net/en/5050/insight-into-bosnia -and-herzegovinas-male-and-female-survivors-of-wartime-rape/ (accessed January 2019).

Foucault, M. 2008. *The birth of biopolitics: Lectures at the Collège de France, 1978–1979*. New York: Palgrave Macmillan.

Funk, J. and Good N. 2017. *Neizlječena trauma: Rad na ozdravljenju I izgradnji mira u BiH*. Sarajevo: TPO Fondacija.

Gavey, N. 2005. *Just sex: The cultural scaffolding of rape*. Hove and Brighton: Routledge.

Goffman E. 1963. *Stigma: Notes on the management of spoiled identity*. Harmondsworth: Penguin Books.

Hayden, R. 2000. "Rape and rape avoidance in ethno-national conflicts: Sexual violence in liminilized states." *American Anthropologist* 102 (1): 27–41.

Helsinki Watch. 1993. *War crimes in Bosnia-Herzegovina:* New York: Helsinki Watch, a division of Human Rights Watch.

Henry, N. 2010. "The impossibility of bearing witness: Wartime rape and the promise of justice." *Violence against Women* 16 (10): 1098–1119.

Hesford, W. S. 1999. "Reading 'rape stories': Material rhetoric and the trauma of representation." *College English* 62 (2): 192–221.

Husić, S., Šiljak I., Osmanović E., Đekić F., and Heremić L. 2014. *Još uvijek smo žive! Istraživanje o dugoročnim posljedicama ratnog silovanja i strategijama suočavanja preživjelih u Bosni i Hercegovini*. Medica: Zenica.

Jelin, E. 2003. *State repression and the labors of memory*. Minneapolis: University of Minnesota Press.

Kannenberg, R. L. 2003. *Sociotherapy for sociopaths – Resocial group*. Wisconsin: Healthcare Publications.

Kelly, L. 1988. *Surviving sexual violence*. New Jersey: Wiley.

Kidron, C. A. 2009. "Toward an ethnography of silence: The lived presence of the past in the everyday life of holocaust trauma survivors and their descendants in Israel." *Current Anthropology* 50 (1): 5–19.

La Capra, D. 1994. *Representing the holocaust history, theory, trauma*. Ithaca, NY: Cornell University Press.

Laumann, E. O. and Gagnon, J. 1995. *Conceiving sexuality: Approaches to sex research in a postmodern world*. New York: Routledge.

Lewis, L. J. 2006. "Sexuality, race and ethnicity." In R. D. McAnulty and M. M. Burnette (Eds.), *Sex and sexuality* (229–265). Westport, CT: Praeger Publishers.

Leys, R. 2000. *Trauma: A genealogy*. Chicago: University of Chicago Press.

Link, B. and Phelan J. 2014. "Stigma power." *Social Science and Medicine* 103: 24–32.

Lončar, M., Medvedev, V., Jovanović, N., and Hotujac, L. 2006. "Psychological consequences of rape on women in 1991–1995 war in Croatia and Bosnia and Herzegovina." *Croatian Medical Journal* 47 (1): 67–75.

Milroy, H. 2005. *The Western Australian aboriginal child health survey: The social and emotional wellbeing of aboriginal children and young people*. Perth: Curtin University of Technology and Telethon Institute for Child Health Research.

Mookherjee, N. 2006. "Remembering to forget: Public secrecy and memory of sexual violence in the Bangladesh war or 1971." *Journal of Royal Anthropological Institute* 12 (2): 433–450.

Parker, R. and Aggleton, P. 2003. "HIV and AIDS-related stigma and discrimination: A conceptual framework and implications for action." *Social Science & Medicine* 57(1): 13–24.

Pescosolido, B. and Martin, J. 2015. "The Stigma Complex." *Annual Review of Sociology* 41: 87–116.

Phelan, J.C., Link, B.G. and Dovidio, J.F. 2008. "Stigma and prejudice: One animal or two?" *Social Science & Medicine* 67(3): 358–367.

Pilgrim, D. and McCranie, A. 2013. *Recovery and mental health: A critical sociological account*. Basingstoke, UK: Palgrave Macmillan.

Plummer, K. 1995. *Telling sexual stories: Power, change and social worlds*. New York: Routledge.

Quinn, D. M. and Chaudoir, S. R. 2009. "Living with a concealable stigmatized identity: The impact of anticipated stigma, centrality, salience, and cultural stigma on psychological distress and health." *Journal of Personality and Social Psychology* 97: 634–651.

Richters, A., Rutayisire, T., and Dekker, C. 2010. "Care as a turning point in sociotherapy: Remaking the moral world in post-genocide Rwanda." *Medische Antropologie* 22 (1): 93–108.

Ruff-O'Herne, J. 2008. *50 years of silence*. London: William Heinemann.

Sayce, L. 1998. "Stigma, discrimination and social exclusion: What's in a word." *Journal of Mental Health* 7 (4): 331–343.

Schudson, M. 1997. "Lives, laws, and language: Commemorative versus non-commemorative forms of effective public memory." *Communication Review* 2 (1): 3–17.

Seifert, R. 1994. "War and rape: A preliminary analysis." In A. Stiglmayer (Ed.), *Mass rape: The war against women in Bosnia-Herzegovina* (54–72). Lincoln: University of Nebraska Press.

Simon, W. and Gagnon, J. H. 1986. "Sexual scripts: Permanence and change." *Archives of Sexual Behavior* 15 (2): 97–120.

Skjelsbaek, I. 2006. "Therapeutic work with victims of sexual violence in war and postwar: A discourse analysis of Bosnian experiences." *Peace and Conflict Journal of Peace Psychology* 12 (2): 93–118.

Skjelsabek, I. 2011. *The political psychology of war rape: Studies from Bosnia-Herzegovina*. New York: Routledge.

Smart, L. and Wegner, D. 1999. "Covering up what can't be seen: Concealable stigma and mental control." *Journal of Personality and Social Psychology* 77 (3): 474–486.

Smith, A. 2005. *Conquest: Sexual violence and American Indian genocide*. Boston: South End Press.

Sontag, S. 2003. *Regarding the pain of others*. New York: Picador.

Taussig, M. 1999. *Defacement: Public secrecy and the labor of the negative*. San Francisco: Stanford University Press.

Tyler, I. 2013. *Revolting subjects: Social abjection and resistance in neoliberal Britain*. London: Zed.

Tyler, I. and Slater, T. 2018. "Rethinking the sociology of stigma." *The Sociological Review Monographs* 66 (4): 721–743.

Ullman, S. E. 2010. *Talking about sexual assault: Society's response to survivors*. Washington, DC: American Psychological Association.

UNFPA. 2016. Stigma against survivors of conflict related sexual violence in Bosnia and Herzegovina – Research Summary. Available: https://ba.unfpa.org/sites/default/files/pub-pdf/UNFPA%20Stigma%20Short%20ENG%20FIN1_0.pdf (accessed 9 December 2019).

Vincent, B. and Durham, H. 2014. "Sexual violence in armed conflict: From breaking the silence to breaking the cycle." *International Review of the Red Cross* 96 (894): 427–434.

Vinitzky-Seroussi, V. and Teeger, C. 2010. "Unpacking the unspoken: Silence in collective memory and forgetting." *Social Forces* 88 (3): 1103–1122.

Vojnović, V. 2006. "Ne plači, bona, seno!." Available at http://www.popbo ks.com/artic le/2849 (accessed December 2017).

Vranić, S. 1996. *Breaking the wall of silence: The voices of raped Bosnia*. Zagreb: Izdanja Antibarbarus.

Wacquant, L. 2008. *Urban outcasts: A comparative sociology of advanced marginality*. Cambridge: Polity.

Waterston, A. and Rylko-Bauer, B. 2006. "Out of the shadows of history and memory: Personal family narratives in ethnographies of rediscovery." *American Ethnologist* 33 (3): 397–412.

Waynryb, R. 2001. *The silence: How tragedy shapes talk*. St Leonard's, N.S.W.: Allen & Unwin.

White, H. 1992. "Historical emplotment and the problem of truth." In S. Friedlander (Ed.), *Probing the limits of representation: Nazism and the 'final solution'* (37–53). Cambridge, MA: Harvard University Press.

Whiteley, J. S. 1986. "Sociotherapy and psychotherapy in the treatment of personality disorder: Discussion paper." *Journal of the Royal Society of Medicine* 79: 721–725.

Whittier, D. K. and Simon, W. 2001. "The fuzzy matrix of 'My Type' in intrapsyhsic sexual scripting." *Sexualities* 4 (2): 139–165.

Wiseman, H. and Barber, J. P. 2008. *Echoes of the trauma: Relational themes and emotions in chilren of holocaust survivors*. Cambridge: Cambridge University Press.

Zerubavel, E. 2010. "The social sound of silence: Toward a sociology of denial." In Ben-Ze'ev Efrat and Jay Winter (Eds.), *Shadows of war: A social history of silence in the twentieth century* (32–44). Cambridge: Cambridge University Press.

4 Mothering with the trauma of war rape

(Il)legitimate motherhoods

In mid-June 2018, several associations around Bosnia-Herzegovina gathered to raise awareness about putting an end to conflict-related sexual violence and to share solidarity with the victims and survivors of rapes committed during the 1990s war. The crowd, consisting mostly of survivors and supporters from the region, was not large. Yet one could detect a gradual increase in public and media participation since 2015, when the United Nations General Assembly proclaimed June 19 as The International Day for the Elimination of Sexual Violence in Conflict. Just a little less than a month later, in mid-July, a few thousand people from all around the world came to honor the victims of the Srebrenica genocide and to offer support to those surviving mothers who had lost their sons during the mass killings.

Although not specifically stated, mothers were among the rape survivors at the first gathering; similarly, there were rape survivors among mothers in the second. But strangely enough – or perhaps not – these two occasions, or commemorations, did not deal with the legacy of war crimes from an intersectional perspective. Postwar identity and the subsequent idea of the collective memory of women rape survivors are connected to *the very act of the war crime* – that is, war-related rape and sexual violence. This connection nurtures the idea that this act labels them as *war-rape survivors*. The women, mothers survivors from Srebrenica built their survivorship *on assigned social roles*, particularly and sometimes exclusively around the images of (traditional) motherhood. What is common to both groups is that their individual stories and experiences blend together to form a collective narrative that becomes a more or less coherent unit. But the cultural memory that has been built around modes of memorizing and the consequences that those women live with in today's postconflict Bosnia-Herzegovina praise either the ideal, traditional motherhood of women genocide survivors or the innocent victimhood of women rape survivors. In terms of collective memory, these two narratives barely intersect.

The narrative is different when it comes to motherhood, nationalism, and war. The use of female bodies for very specific political purposes in furthering war's

nationalistic agendas has been largely addressed and discussed in past studies
(Papić 1994; Korac 1998; Žarkov 2007). Not only have geographical territories
and nations been framed in discourses of motherhood (for a critical examination,
see Žarkov 1995; Nikolić-Ristanović 2000), according to some scholars, such
prewar symbolism and gendered metaphors determined the ideological premise
for employing sexualized violence during the war in Bosnia-Herzegovina. Once
women's identities became tied to their reproductive responsibilities for the purposes of the war, it became hard to distinguish between the languages of motherhood, nationalism, and war (Bracewell 1996; Yuval-Davis 1997; Pankov et al.
2011). Those dynamics, according to Patricia Albanese, impacted the renewal of
an archaized social environment, "a culture that attempts to resurrect institutionalized traditional gender relations and thereby relegitimize patriarchal domination"
(Albanese 2001, 1004). The war being fought through bodies operates with odd
and contradictory identity politics in which women are simultaneously heroines
and victims. A "patriotic mother," or the "ever-ready womb for war" (Åhäll 2012,
106) portray women as weapons because of their ability to produce new fighters.
At the same time, however, her biology makes her the primary target of attempts
to either destroy her reproductive capacity or to completely instrumentalize that
capacity through forced impregnation. These politics were essential in the formation of patriarchal narratives of victims and/or survivors – of womanhood itself
– after the war. It also often affected the ways in which women lent their support
in postwar reconstruction efforts, especially among fellow women (Walsh 1997;
Kleck 2006; Mulalic 2011).

While many women were distressed by their own traumatic experiences in
the aftermath of the war, social expectations compelled them to focus on the
reconstruction of their homes and on serving their shattered families before they
could deal with their own psychological and physical recoveries (Danopoulos,
Skandalis & Isakovic 2012, 145). These expectations are based on traditional
understandings of women as mothers, either in the literal sense or as carrying out
maternal tasks as nurturers and caregivers. Many studies, particularly those conducted by feminist scholars, have attempted to deconstruct this in theory; empirically, however, most households outside of urban centers still largely practice
very traditional forms of family and gender relations/roles. To be able to cope
with the chaos of postwar social realities, traditional, ethnic, religious, and gender
identities are often revitalized to glorify the past, evoking "neo-traditional beliefs
in a purported 'golden age' of patriarchal social rule" (Schnabel & Tabyshalieva
2012, 17). In this sense, the experience of Bosnian civilians is not much different.
Despite recent developments in the field of gender and sexuality, the conservative
postwar backlash and "social archaization" (Albanese 2001, 1008) have certainly
manifested at all levels of everyday life, taking a sharp turn from previous, relatively liberal gender politics and Westernized women's movements in Yugoslavia
(Pusić 1976; Papić 1979; Kašić et al. 2012).

Archaic patterns of gender discrimination and patriarchal rule in the aftermath
of the war are easily found, specifically in the creation of the socially desired
collective memory of women survivors. A tendency to place their testimonies

inside the victimhood narrative has led to an extremely limited and problematic knowledge of survivors' postwar recovery, which reflect only a highly gendered and victimized identities (Simić 2012; Močnik 2017). In a way, the repetitive representations of traditional motherhood and womanhood are employed to make the horrendous crimes believable and the offenders responsible. But in a subtler sense, such representations also confirm the very paradigm of rape culture, in which a woman – always a suspect in a rape allegation – is considered to have invited the rape by her appearance or behavior. To be deserving of the status of victim and be respected as such, she must respond to the prescribed societal hegemonic norms of womanhood, which are also very often linked to her skills as a mother.

Women's experiences of motherhood after they experienced something as traumatic as war and war rape, is almost completely overshadowed by these narrow analytical lenses, through which women are viewed between the politics of nationalism and gender as such. Rarely in the past research, one could learn more about mothers who had children before they were raped, those who bore children from war rapes, and those who gave birth after being raped during the war (but not as a result of rape) or in its aftermath. For numerous women, the impact of war on motherhood is "to have one's breasts chopped off" (Gallimore 2017, 14), a metaphor that expresses the pain of the psychological and physical destruction of a woman's body *as a maternal body* deprived of the opportunity for motherhood (Zraly, Rubin, & Mukaman 2013). In her report for the Balkan Investigating Report Network, Elameri Škrgić Mikulić includes an excerpt from her interview with a war-rape survivor, who explains this deprivation as, "Yes, they took my unborn child. The truth is that I could never become a mother, I could never be and I am not a mother" (in Škrgić Mikulić 2016).

Motherhood, which is defined by so many individual women in the aftermath of the war, in very different ways both personally and socially, has been addressed inadequately by previous scholarship. Some survivors have (re)started families and raised children after the war, and today, many have already seen their grandchildren grow and mature. Yet there remains a shortfall of ethnographic evidence and inadequate analytical insight into their experiences, which usually has its origins in their fear of social ostracism, stigmatization, and shame in the event of disclosure (Ahrens 2006; Skjelsbaek 2006; Weiss 2010). From my own experience in the field, it is striking how strongly women desire to separate their war-rape experience from their children and the general practice of mothering, even though that mothering may lead to a place of healing, not only as a result of *giving birth* to new life, but also in *being reborn* themselves in this new role, which is accompanied by a new mission. Most of the survivors with whom I have worked would agree that being a mother was often their only hope for continuing to pursue personal healing and social reintegration. One of the mother's statements illustrates this:

If not for her /daughter/ I am not sure if I would still be alive. But when she was born, and this was in 1997, I was only thinking about her. When I got dark thoughts or my pain was too great, I only thought of her and I could push myself through. I am not sure I would survive if I were not blessed with her.

(M57, Central Bosnia)

Many of the conversations that I overheard in the associations where survivors gather were about their children and grandchildren. Those who used social media would also post mostly very emotional and loving pictures of their (grand)children. Yet, as much as these mothers emphasized the importance of their offspring to their survival, they would also mention the importance of maintaining a distance between the (grand)children and their traumatic past.

The division between the two identities – one of a survivor and another one of a mother – became especially apparent to me when, in the library of the Cure Foundation in Sarajevo during the summer of 2019, I was reviewing feminist publications on grassroots gender and antiwar activism in the region. I became aware that these readings contained very few intersections between motherhood, feminist activism, and war rapes. While the many editions of "Zbornik Žene u crnom," for instance, followed a precise feminist-activist framework, none of those activists who were (are) also mothers had at any point reflected upon raising their own children in a patriarchally hostile environment, mentioning neither their own role nor their personal experiences. The very personal narrative of mothering in times of war, postwar, and general patriarchal rule and how it affects them in a very private sphere, was, strangely, invisible. As there would be a need for these women to follow two separate lives – to keep the safety of her home private and unknown to readers and to fully assume her role in street activism and antiwar movements.

I tried to reach out to some of these activists – mothers who were particularly active and vocal in the antiwar demonstrations of 1990 – I was unfortunately unsuccessful. This has left me with assumptions rather than conclusions, but also with further thoughts as to how one might understand the domestic lives and relationships of mothers and their children as primal peace education. Incorporating the diverse postwar experiences of mothering, particularly after surviving atrocities such as rape, has the potential to break down the patriarchal expectations and social demands associated with the continuation of traditional romanticized and asexualized motherhood, I assumed. Yet, the absence of evidence on mothering after surviving war rape supports the narrative of pure mothers, and her sexuality is inexistent (except in relation to its reproductive role). Once a woman is socially perceived as sexually disgraced, as happens in the case of war-rape survivors, her capacity for becoming an appreciated and respected mother is neglected.

Today's gendered narratives as they exist in the collective memory most often classify women as powerless and defenseless victims (Leydesdorff 2007; Cogan 2013; Jacobs 2017). If motherhood is present in these narratives, then it is in the form of *suffering mothers*, in a traditional, patriarchally designed motherhood that is full of sacrifice and devotion but lacks the real presence of the woman herself. Her existence is contingent on the well-being of her beloved ones, children, and spouse. To approach these dynamics, I analyze postwar notions of mother-hood and mothering through the prism of an *undisclosed motherhood* (among mother–survivors of war rape) put into comparative perspective with *tragic comfort-discomfort motherhood* (with the example of mother–survivors of gen-dercide[1] in Srebrenica). A very particular representation of Srebrenica's "moth-ers of all mothers" – strongly representing the ideal, traditional, and patriarchal images of mothers and motherhood – slowly overshadowed the testimonies and experiences of mother–survivors from other regions who experienced different yet still-shattering atrocities during the war. In terms of motherhood, women who survived the crimes of rape and sexual violence became particularly mar-ginalized. If they appear as "mothers" in direct connection with their war-rape experience, it is usually through the voices of their (abandoned) children born of rape. Recently we can follow up on the increased public presence of, and interest in, children born of rape. As those children have become increasingly vocal and have adopted approaches to the topic that differ from those used previously by survivors, they can also help to form new narratives and representations of their mother–survivors.

Over the years, public appearances by members of the Mothers of the Enclaves of Srebrenica and Žepa (henceforth, "The Association") became recognized glob-ally as the unquestionable, fixed, and sacred archetype and ideal of devoted and loving mothers, patiently carrying the burden of the painful loss of beloved fam-ily members, particularly their sons. Like many other women's group activities after the war, their struggle confirms affirmative gender essentialism (Djurić-Kuzmanović et al. 2008, 276) through positive images of women as nurturers and peacemakers. Following the Srebrenica massacre, members of The Association found their greatest strength in performing their roles as mothers – not only as mothers of their own sons, but of everyone who suffered through the slaughter. Olivera Simić (2009, 229) notes how

> they [members of The Association] employ their reproductive role in a social
> context, thus representing themselves as the mothers of *all people* who died
> in the Srebrenica genocide. They are the mothers to their sons, but also to
> their husbands, relatives and neighbors, since they embrace them all as their
> "lost children" under their motherhood claim.

Unlike the prewar ideological constructions, these women are not only the *body of the nation*; they have become the *body of the nation that survived*. In this process, their performance is purified, regulated, and almost completely desexualized. As such, they are "invisibly visible as a symbolic fantasy" (Einstein 1996, 54). To achieve their goal, they are omnipresent at public gatherings, marches, and media events, but are generally *not seen* as individuals, and especially not as women out-side of their social roles as mothers (Simić 2009, 229) and as agents in search of the truth. The discourse that defines them as mother–survivors frames their testi-monies; consequently, it shapes the knowledge we have (or lack) about their own war experiences. The search for those who disappeared and were killed, therefore, overshadows the testimonies of those who survived. When The Association does appear in public, its members talk about others. As is expected from ideal mothers, their stories are pushed to the margins while they care for their loved ones, searching for their remains and telling their stories. In this way, they maintain the patriarchal order of women who operate only in the sphere of domestic, private life.

To enter into male-operated public arenas, they speak *on behalf* of their male relatives, their *killed males*. The main story is thus no longer about women survivors, but about women survivors who embody their murdered male counterparts in order to tell their stories. When they do come forward to share their own experiences, those stories are rarely about sexual violence, which leads one to believe that the absence of rape stories in Srebrenica is a direct consequence of how mothers navigate their naturalized private spaces – with the need to come to the fore only to speak in the name of, and for the faith of, their male relatives. How come that the representations of mothers of the killed and vanished children so rarely mentioned their experiences of war-inflicted (sexualized) violence, to the extent that one can easily conjure up memories of the Srebrenica massacre in terms of a complete absence of the memorialization of women victims of rape and sexualized violence (Jacobs 2017, 432)?

Srebrenica has gained recognition as a site of genocide, but any violence other than extermination (of men) is rarely discussed. At the same time, a few scholars (Copelon 1995; Allen 1996; Russel-Brown 2003) have discussed the sexual violence committed against Muslim women in Bosnia through the lens of genocidal rape, but almost never with reference to Srebrenica. War rape and sexual violence in the context of Srebrenica and gendercide are generally poorly evidenced (for some evidence, see Human Rights Watch Report 1995; Ahmetašević 2010), although there has recently been more attention paid specifically to sexual violence perpetrated by the United Nations Protection Force (UNPROFOR) peacekeepers and humanitarian aid workers both before and after the massacre (Bowcott 2005, Bolkovac & Lynn 2011; PBS 2018). While exploring my interest in sexual violence in Srebrenica, I mentioned some of the recent debates around UNPROFOR's involvement in these crimes to a survivor, who responded with a story of how she was offered comfort by a "male companion" while asking for a wood stove:

> I came to the office, where you could put your name on the list and ask for some basic appliances. As winter was approaching and I wanted to cook my own food, I asked for the wood stove. The humanitarian worker who was in charge of communicating with me told me that unfortunately I can't get one, but he can come to my bed and warm me up with his hairy body. I didn't want to keep quiet so I hissed at him: I would take you instead of the wood stove, but you can only warm me up from one side at once; the other side of my body will still be freezing cold.
>
> (K, June 2018, Sarajevo)

After listening to this story, I asked her if she had heard of similar experiences from other women, or if she could connect me with members of The Association who were, to her knowledge, also testifying against crimes of sexual violence. She immediately directed me to the Association of Women Victims of War, the largest organization in Sarajevo dealing with legal and bureaucratic support to survivors, saying:

> We heard that rapes are happening, and it is a crime, like any other. But this is not what we focus on here. After rape you can recover. You can go for healing. We are not searching for healing because this is not injury; what we deal with here is not injured women or men, but dead men. You can't heal this.
>
> (K, Sarajevo 2018)

We spent almost three more hours discussing the events in Srebrenica. It was very challenging for me to keep the conversation focused on the legacy of war rapes and to gather more information on mother–survivors who had been sexually violated. When at the end of our conversation I thanked her for her time, I tried once more to emphasize that I would still appreciate it if she came across any mothers raped who would be willing to contact me. She gave me the name and phone number of a woman who had recently disclosed to her daughter that she had been raped. She added:

> Oh, but she is from //name of the town omitted//. But she was raped. I don't want to sound like we don't have women in our organization who did not survive rapes. It is just not our goal to deal with these problems. This is why they go to Women Victims of War, to testify and to register. In our organization, we are mothers who lost their sons, and the truth of this is what is important for us. We don't really deal with what kind of crimes were committed; what is important is that our people disappeared, and our lives were ruined.
>
> (K, 2018, Sarajevo)

After the visit, I once again read the mission statement of The Association on their web page, and it clearly stated that their goal is "to gather survivors and family members of the victims who disappeared in 1995" (Udruženje 'Pokret Majke enclave Srebrenica I Žepa' 2017). It also stated that The Association was established out of the *need for mothers* to find out about their missing family members. Although I examined other materials available on their web page, I found only one specific reference to war rape, which noted that The Association was one of the co-organizers of the 2012 Mass Rapes as War Strategy Conference.[2] The Association, of course, does not represent all survivors of the Srebrenica massacre. As a matter of fact, it is rather exclusive in terms of its membership. However, their work and presence gained extremely powerful recognition and sociopolitical influence, which pushes to the periphery a number of other narratives that do not affirm their story. In July 2018, during my stay in Srebrenica, I had the opportunity to engage in an informal conversation with three mother–widows, none of whom were members of The Association. Only one of the women responded directly to my question about rapes:

> I was not raped myself, but I heard rapes were happening. I have never seen or talked to a woman who was raped, but I believe them. Thank god, this did not happen to me. But if you survived this, and after you gave birth, you raised new life, so it is easy to forget. You can live on. War happened but is now over. What could I do after all my family was killed? I only search for them; this is what I do. And I buried my only son back in 2008. Can I live on now? Maybe if I was thirty, who knows, but I am sixty-seven now, I can't start my life again.
>
> (S, Srebrenica 2018)

Members of The Association perform the culturally appropriate and accepted roles of mothers – moreover, they are always carefully covered with their traditional head scarves and photographed in front of their reconstructed houses, in their flower gardens, or among nishan-tombstones. By representing the "embodiment of moral authority *par excellence*" (Burchianti 2004, 142), The Association joined the global movement of mothers whose motherhood overcame the rhetoric of maternal suffering to become a visible and powerful form of political struggle. But in order to preserve the socially comforting images of traditional motherhood that appear in the official narrative, The Association largely omits and dismisses notes on rape crimes. The Association's influence is far-reaching, and so we can only speculate as to how this affects the narratives of other mothers. Continuous exposure to the narrative of the importance to remember Srebrenica massacre, makes it easy to fall under the influence of the preferred format of tragic motherhood.

By ignoring the intersectional (ab)use of war identities in which women are targeted on the basis of their gender, sexuality, and ethnic and religious affiliation, tragic motherhood offers mother–survivors from Srebrenica *comfort-discomfort* memorialization. While it is *uncomfortable* to live the life of a widowed mother who has lost every family member, it is still more *comfortable* than living with the stigma of rape and being ostracized by living family members. But women who have suffered during war can lose their children as mothers and suffer from rape. Despite being raped and losing their children during the war, some women later became mothers again. Representatives of The Association prefer those aspects of their gendered identity that would help them to advance their struggle for justice. The tragic mother is an archetypal figure who does not demand that society change its established, prewar hegemonic practices. Accepting the legacy of rape and sexual violence among survivors that became mothers in the aftermath of the war, on the other hand, demands unlearning some essential social agreements, dynamics, and power systems.

If the ideal postwar motherhood of mothers from Srebrenica is usually asexualized and alienated from sexual crimes, women rape survivors from other regions often privatize their motherhood experience completely and separate it from their public battles. If there is silence regarding rape among the mothers of Srebrenica, we can identify a similar pattern in the case of motherhood among survivors of rapes. In their testimonies and public appearances, motherhood is mentioned only occasionally, and never fully exposed. The narrative of the collective memory of mothers who are war-rape survivors includes primarily victimhood narratives but also narratives of silence and marginalization. While the mothers of Srebrenica would like to speak to their dead children, survivors of rape fear breaking the silence because their children would hear them. However, mother–survivors of rapes mostly agreed that it would be important to share their history with their children, provided both – children and mothers would be somehow prepared to avoid ostracism, abandonment, stigma, or fear of spreading interethnic and inter-religious hatred among their children or their children's friends (notes from work-shop, 2018, Northeast Bosnia).

A survivor, born into and later married into a mixed marriage, shared that her grandson has friends of different ethnic backgrounds. She did not oppose these friendships, nor did she perceive children from other ethnic backgrounds as "the dangerous Other." However, she fears that these relationships would suffer should her daughters, who know about her rape story, share this with her grandson:

> I would like him to know. And I believe that one day, when he becomes older, he will find my story and he will know what to do with it. I also believe that he has a good heart and that my story will not affect his friendships.
>
> (H68, Northeast Bosnia 2018)

Conversations with survivors revealed only a partial interest in disclosure, mostly due to the belief that sharing these stories would relieve them of the burden of the crimes. One mother shared with me her fear that disclosing her status as a rape survivor to her children would cast a shadow over her role as a mother:

> I feel my kids love me. I feel they can feel how much I love them. But I fear if I tell them, they will only see me as rape survivor. But how will they see me? I can't even imagine what they will see! I want to be a mother for them, a good mother, and this is the only thing I want.
>
> (A, Northeast Bosnia 2018)

However, many of the survivors I spoke with believed that disclosure would make sense only if their children were to accept the truth of their stories without doubt or opposition, and only if their relationships following the disclosure would not suffer. Two survivors mentioned that disclosing to their children helped them to break their silence and come to terms with their past. When I raised the issue of the importance of the gender of their children – both women were the mothers of daughters only – the entire group agreed that it is harder to speak with sons than with daughters. One of the survivors reports:

> There is this connection [between her and her daughter]. We have the same biological body. We talk about menstruation and we joke about sex. Talking

about sex with her is no problem. But you can't do this if you have a son. Men look at these things differently. One just can't talk in the same way with women and men.

(A47, Northeast Bosnia 2018)

Her opinion opened up a chaotic conversation that was challenging to facilitate and which led to several disagreements about the extent to which society is patriarchal and how raising children depends on how their gender influences their relationships later in life. Survivors mentioned that the family background and their marital status is an important factor when it comes to decision either to speak up or not. For example, two public representatives from two organizations that help rape survivors are unmarried and childless. A representative from another organization and her daughter share the direct experience of having been raped in each other's presence. In conversations with survivors, it was clear that family relationships are important aggravating circumstances when it comes to the question of disclosure.

One of the survivors with whom I spoke regularly appears in court and has participated in open public events several times, including the Foča commemoration of 2018. As unexpected events in the city prevented us from meeting, we had a brief telephone conversation in July 2018, during which she told me that no one in her family knows about her history, including her husband and her two children, both of whom were born after the war. She never felt strong enough to disclose. As her name or face can now be found in news reports of the events she has attended, I asked her whether she fears being recognized by her family. She answered:

> My husband is not interested, and he is always trying to get away if I mention anything about the war. I doubt he will ever find anything. I think he knows anyway, but he just works so hard to suppress everything. Even if he sees my face on TV, I think he will just pretend and say nothing. As for my kids… maybe my activism is now my way to disclose without disclosing. Maybe I am hoping that this is how my kids can learn about me, without directly saying anything. And if they ask me, I will always tell them everything. But only if they ask me.

(M49, Central Bosnia 2018)

Perhaps paying too much attention to the assumed universal pattern of survivor's silence has deterred us from exploring other important social factors. One important question often left out in the past is how to address those family members of survivors who are ill-informed and ill-prepared. While many survivors who are willing to participate in research have undergone long-term therapeutic processes and have engaged with professional support and connected to other survivors, their family members, especially their husbands, have only rarely been engaged in the same or similar systematic healing and recovery processes. As I understand and investigate the trauma of war rape as a social – and not only a psychological

– phenomenon, I do not believe that the stigma associated with those events and their legacy can be broken only by survivors who work through their trauma in some sort of individualized, medicalized, and psychotherapeutic process.

Most of the survivors who are married and/or have children told me that they have difficulty disclosing to their families. Because they have heard from others who have been abandoned, some do not disclose simply because they do not have the strength and motivation to do so. One survivor disclosed to her three daughters upon returning home:

> It's now been almost 8 years. They still don't believe me. I am very persistent. I tried many times. One of my daughters, the middle one, she thinks I am crazy and that I lie. She, no, all three, they don't believe that any of these things really happened. They don't believe me. I know these women are saying that it is important to tell our children. I did. But they would just not listen to me.
>
> (M62, Northeast Bosnia 2018)

Many in this same group would agree that the war is now far removed and that they want their children to live in a peaceful society, unencumbered by the past. One mother said that nothing would change for the better if she were to disclose to her children. She added that it was important for her to join a group and share her story with other survivors. On a side note, it was very interesting to observe the constructive response from the group – they expressed that they are willing to travel to other regions of the country to testify and share their stories in front of young people they do not know. For some of them, this idea came to be seen as a compromise between the impossibility of disclosure to their own children and the need to disseminate information and knowledge about the events to teach new generations. In this way, they can still embrace the principles of *mothering* to children, though not necessarily with their own biological children.

The question of disclosing in this way becomes a question of *legitimate motherhood*: a good mother cannot be a raped mother; her devotion, love, and care are not compatible with violence, anger, and trauma. In the narratives we have today, we can see that mothers whose sons were killed are mothers who respond to the normative social rules. Mothers who gave birth as a result of rape have long suffered the greatest stigma, as the memory of rape becomes manifest in a child who some decided to keep. However, the relatively new association, Forgotten Children of War, has in a short time since their establishment in 2015 contributed noticeably to bettering the status of mothers as well as children born of war. Members of the association have been integral in both raising awareness concerning the status of children born of rape and in breaking the stigma related to their mothers. As well, in collaboration with other social actors (for instance through the performance *U ime oca*), members of Forgotten Children of War offer a very new narrative approach, delivered with a much more optimistic and determined attitude compared to what one witnessed in years past.

While those mothers who birthed children from rape are, with the help of their vocal children, considered heroines, those women who survived rape and became mothers only some years after the war remain behind the scenes of public attention. All those representations of mother–survivors suggest that both sexuality and motherhood remain controlled by patriarchal notions, in which the codes of traditional motherhood predispose the sexuality of mothers to assuming a (sexually) submissive role, and where sexuality mostly serves reproduction purposes. If our society does not acknowledge mothers who are war-rape survivors, it can imply that those women should be held responsible for their "lost" motherhood. In a traditional heteronormative society, the label of survivors of war rape not only makes these women unmarriageable, it condemns them as *un-mother-able*. Narratives concerning the collective memory of war-rape survivors help us to socially criminalize and condemn mother–survivors; once they become publicly active and politically present, their motherhood status, their *struggle for survival as mothers*, somehow vanishes.

The nonexistence of motherhood experience in the testimonies of survivors suggests that society is not ready to connect what is now perceived as "polluted, dirty sexuality" with what we still praise as sacred, "pure" motherhood. On the other hand, this same demand creates the artificial and unrealistic portrayal of mother–survivors of the Srebrenica gendercide as asexualized: women whose sexuality was meant only for creating a new human being, only to be then brutally murdered. Regardless of the types of crimes they survived, all women are continuously subjected to discursive and symbolical violence under patriarchal rule – they are expected to stay in this role even when deprived of their actual motherhood, as in the case of the mothers of Srebrenica. They are expected to live this role not only within the confines of their family now that the whole world is watching and judging their mothering capabilities. And this is perhaps the biggest tragedy of their motherhood: their *mothering-of-dead-children*, the most profound expression of a true mother's love, somehow makes them role models. On the other hand, the experience of war rape will never allow survivors to become overtly (publicly) satisfied, proud mothers. The stigma of those women will never be broken as long as we refuse to accept the intersections of their identities and to make motherhood after (war) rape socially legitimate.

While most of the mothers who survived Srebrenica who have committed themselves to a lifetime of mourning are not able to speak to their disappeared and murdered children and grandchildren, rape survivors – who became mothers after the war – would be able to share their stories if we were to create spaces where such narratives were normalized and accepted. I was surprised to witness so much willingness and optimism in a response to the idea to engage in an intergenerational dialogue together with a postwar youth. At the same time, I could confirm through my youth work that we are now working with a generation which – thanks perhaps to greater access to information via online platforms – is cognitively and emotionally mature enough, and which is now sufficiently distanced from the war, to listen to survivors and to help break the silence. Together with the survivors, we started to shape the idea, how young people from different regions

– not necessarily the (biological) children and grandchildren of survivors – could contribute to breaking the silence by comforting mother–survivors, allowing them to talk about both their motherhood and their (abused) sexuality. In this way, mother–survivors could "rehearse the disclosure" with other young people before coming face to face with their own (grand)children.

There is a vicious circle of disappointments in survivors' expectations, in which justice for most survivors is not realized and where political denial persists. In a similar fashion, society (un)consciously contributes to the further stigmatization and marginalization of women by supporting traditional gender roles, which are manifested as silence, obedience, and looking after one's own needs only after the needs of one's family members have been met. However, in this cycle, the possibility of dialogue between survivors and the next generation provides an optimistic – although not yet fully explored – grassroots approach to fighting stigma, nurturing understanding, and challenging quite radically the existing collective memory that perpetuates unequal gender codes and harmful and violent sexualities.

Teaching trauma-free sexual scripts in traumatized homes

According to Chodorov, a daughter's identification with the mother starts in infancy and continues throughout childhood, and while the mother anticipated future motherhood, the daughter is prepared to create, care for, and maintain a family (Chodorow 1978, 167). On the other hand, the role model for boys – that is, a father – is often absent in patriarchal societies, which prepares a boy to be "the Other": not the mother, but one separated, different from her. This, claims Chodorow (1978, ibid.), excludes him from the private sphere of the home, pushes him away, and prepares him for the competitive and aggressive world outside of the comfortable closeness of the family. Fifty years later, when our knowledge of the variety of genders and sexualities has been largely circulated and increasingly accepted and recognized in different sociopolitical contexts, this dualistic dichotomy seems outdated and dangerous.

A reconceptualization of the practice of gender essentialism seems crucial in challenging the patriarchal conception of personal identities and roles and for peace theory (Duhan Kaplan 1994, 169). Together with other feminist thinkers, such as Karen J. Warren (1990), Duhan Kaplan problematized celebrating the caretaker archetype in connection to peacebuilding. The gender-stereotyped image, in which the woman takes care of the family, nurtures and maintains loving relationships, and balances unstable dynamics, reinforces the same systems of oppression that subjected her to the violent and abusive experiences of the war. Women serving others cannot lead to sustainable peace, claim those theories: dismantling "all systems and structures of domination and subordination, and the psychological and conceptual forces that keep them in place" is necessary to create and sustain a long-lasting, future peace (Duhan Kaplan 1994, 170).

While acknowledging that acceptance of patriarchal role divisions is outdated and dangerous, I want to think of the ethnographic field as a living and everchanging habitus that will not necessarily follow the same path as theoretical criticism. In addition, the criticism on a discursive level can nevertheless be still maintained through actions. For instance, while many women today acknowledge the everyday oppression and toxicity of patriarchal systems, they keep acting according to its rules, both psychologically (individually, unconsciously) and sociologically (collectively, consciously) to maintain their (subordinate) positions in this very system. This is not to point to anyone, but rather to bring to the fore the stubborn reality of the empirical world, which is sometimes overshadowed by progressive aspirations elaborated upon in theoretical communities.

For most of the survivors who collaborated with me in this study, transferring traditional, binary gender roles and traditional, "decent" understandings and uses of sexuality to their offspring is a matter of pride and successful mothering. Raising her daughters to be smart and independent but also "marriageable," and their boys to be respectful but also caring, is something these mothers aspire to; it would also confirm that their mothering has been successful and accomplished. However, as many survivors conform to traditional gender norms and affirm the place of sexuality as private (and for girls, also silent and unspoken), the country and the region of Western Balkans in general is undergoing general social changes in this respect, as is any other place in the globalized world. Information and education about sexuality and gender is now available to young people, and informal activities and events are organized regularly to work against toxic femininities/masculinities, nonbinary gender understanding, and diverse sexualities. Various nongovernmental organizations, such as the aforementioned CURE, are extremely vocal – and also effective – in raising awareness and providing informal education concerning sexuality and gender. In addition, the omnipresence of digital media has extended sex education far beyond the home and institutional schooling. And in many cases, I would say, for the better.

Survivors believe that the experience of war rape teaches us to "resist the traditional," particularly in breaking the silence among women – those raped during the war, but also those beaten up in their everyday home lives, and those harassed in the workplace. What we can learn is a lecture on consent: knowledge of marital rape and normalized domestic and sexual violence both before and in the aftermath of war. These are the premises that survivors put on the table when I came up with the idea of visiting a school to engage with the teenagers in a conversation about the consequences of war rape and its take-aways for today's generations. This encounter was inspiring and educational for all of us in many ways, but mostly because it highlighted many obvious divergences that are the result of intergenerational differences. A workshop was organized in 2018 – a collaboration between one of the associations for war-rape survivors and a local school – yet at the request of the survivors we visited a school that was in a different region quite far away from their home town.

The meeting was the result of many conversations, one of which included a discussion about the possibility of having the survivors talk with the youth in such a way that it would help the survivors "rehearse" how they would communicate their stories to their own children later on. Another introduced the idea of better incorporating survivors into peace education conducted with young people. The third one involved the survivors' belief that they must share their first-hand experiences with the children to teach them a "history lesson." For the participating children, however, the main purpose of the workshop was to meet the survivors in person and to learn about their experiences directly, to be able to ask questions and to engage in collective brainstorming as to how those experiences should be communicated in the current sociopolitical context. Both sides were excited, and although it was an intense experience to witness the stories, both survivors and students left the event feeling rather motivated and positive.

At the start of one workshop, one of the participants asked to be identified by their preferred gender pronoun. The two survivors, both aged around 50, found themselves confused, as neither was clear about the meaning of this, especially when some of the participants identified as "them" and another as "two-spirited." Only later, when we were commuting back together, did one of them ask me to clarify the meaning of the multiple genders, and they showed surprise: this was new information for them. They were also surprised, and a little intimidated, that the girls spoke about sex very directly. I wrote in my diary the following day:

> Survivors repeat how important it is to talk directly to the kids about what happened to them. They seem genuinely interested in participating in this kind of workshop. But yesterday's experience made me wonder in what way today's generation can learn "from the history." What is the learning moment? From this concrete example – and I would have to run more workshops to confirm this – I could see a huge (perhaps generational) gap in understanding sexuality. It is true that this school is also a bit different and I might get different feedback elsewhere. Yet, if there is a learning point in the experience of mass rape survivors during the war for today's 16-year olds, what is it?

Evidence of the mass rapes that were committed during the war in Bosnia-Herzegovina has contributed significantly to our current understanding of rape culture, trauma studies, and restorative justice. However, it did not necessarily impact the ideological bent of the survivors' understanding of sexuality and gender or how they see their impact as family breeders. Despite agreeing that rape is the perpetrator's responsibility, not the victim's, they still hesitated in the face of the girls' exaggerated openness. One of the survivors elaborated: "It is not that I am against her [her daughter] being happy and joyful and playful. But we know how this world is. I fear for her. Unfortunately, we live in a society where we cannot trust men."

To a certain degree, war is such an extraordinary event that many youth find it impossible to connect with the survivor's story and transfer its meaning to the current situation. On another occasion, while talking to a group of teenagers and discussing the question of lessons from history, a boy commented that it is just impossible for him "to imagine who can do this type of act." I tried to reverse the story a little bit and asked the girls if they would be afraid should something unexpected happen – say, mass street violence that got out of control. One of the girls said, "I do not fear, but my mother does, she fears for me so much!" and she giggled.

In my workshops on prevention of sexual violence, I often show them the "pyramid of hate" model, which I adjust to frame gender-based and sexual violence. With the help of this model, I try to discuss with them normalized everyday patterns such as sexist jokes, flirting which borders on or is rooted in bullying, and mansplaining. It is usually eye-opening for most of them – how we do not problematize most of these cases but accept them as a normal part of everyday relationship dynamics. At the conclusion, we would usually try to understand how these simple, apparently harmless acts connect to the radical use of sexual violence, as in wars and mass atrocities/mass violence. One of the learning moments for me was this: As a society, we are generally socialized from a very early stage to integrate toxic sexuality; why then are everyday patterns of violent, nonconsensual, and abusive sexuality beyond the pale even for survivors? Once one starts to teach prevention, one begins to recognize obvious, unbalanced power relationships and masochistic and patriarchal patterns in everything. But are these really precursors to "serious" crimes, such as rape? I asked this question mindlessly of my students, whose critical minds turned it into a learning experience. One of the girls responded:

> Every act is serious enough if the person does not give you consent. For this reason I find the form of the "pyramid" misleading. It presupposes hierarchy. Rape is a "serious" crime, and this is why it is at the top. And mansplaining is not, and this is why it is at the bottom.

(S, 2018)

While I agree with her comment, I must also explain that the existing format of the pyramid – where rape is at the top and other types of sexual violence and harassments are found on other levels – does not assume a hierarchy in terms of importance or, as the girl said, "seriousness." It is better understood with the iceberg metaphor, where we usually see the tip but not the portion below the water – a portion that is part of the same, larger problem. Although we focus on learning how to prevent and/or report sexual crimes like rape, we often forget to work on the normalized crimes that lie below the surface. This model elicited very interesting responses when I applied it with the two groups of survivors. For many, this visual display of some very concrete examples of normalized everyday sexual violence (particularly in jokes or stereotypes) offered a new perspective for understanding war rape and their own experiences. At one point, they even started to collect their own stories. One survivor shared how, before the war, she had worked in a café. One of the regular customers – a man from the neighborhood – apparently came to look at her, to gaze at her, and to compliment her. He would always bring her a chocolate or pay for her coffee. Thinking back, she now felt that she never really enjoyed his company, but that she also felt a sense of professional responsibility for this regular customer. When she finished her story, she asked us as a group whether this would now be considered "gender-based violence." As she looked at me, I answered that I understood that she was not enjoying it but felt obliged to respond in this way.

Other survivors started to comment as well, most of them debating whether there is a limit; that if this can be considered violence, then everything can be violence. I do not believe that such cases can ever have a simple conclusion, and there are many details to be taken into consideration, but I found this example particularly illustrative for two reasons. The first is that survivors with personal experience of radical sexual violence – such as rape in wartime – often assume that this experience makes them understand it well. This was very often the reason why the survivors felt that they *had to talk* to the younger generations – to "teach" them and to convey messages about sexual violence. While some survivors lived in abusive relationships or experienced marital rapes prior to the start of the war, they could only recognize it as violence when the war was over; when they learned and understood it alongside their experience of rape in war. For many of the survivors who started to attend sharing circles or any other types of psychosocial support, the process of healing has never solely addressed the process of working through trauma, but included awareness raising and informal modes of sexual and gender education. Some reported that they had never viewed their prewar marriage relationships as abusive, as they simply did not have any knowledge or experiences that differed from their own. "I learned that remaining silent and humble was important for my reputation," says one of my interlocutors,

> but when I joined the circle of survivors, I learned we should not be silent. That this is not about our purity, but about men's crimes. I never talked about sex before the war and I was married and had a child. I only learned to talk about sex when I was told to speak up about my rape experience. I still feel uncomfortable… I believe I should talk with my girl about this, but I don't feel up to it.
>
> (R52, Central Bosnia 2018)

Secondly, recognition of, knowledge about, and prevention of sexual violence are changing immensely. This is not to say that sexual violence is also decreasing, as it is unfortunately not. But we have more reports than before; more reports lead to more evidence; more evidence leads to new practices in prevention; and more prevention leads to more knowledgeable and informed individuals. The very fact that I found myself together with mother–survivors brainstorming on organizing intergenerational workshops on matters of sexual violence in war for the first time, demonstrates that the field is developing and expanding.

However, such workshops and similar programs are for the most part only aspects of informal education; they do not necessarily reach masses of people or general audiences (not only the interested and engaged individuals), they have no regular continuation (which would expose individuals to continuous learning), and they are usually conducted only with young adults (not younger children). For instance, when I suggested that we hold the workshop at a school with youngsters 14–15 years of age, the teacher in charge replied that the topic would be too demanding for such a young audience and the risk (of traumatization or even responses like anger and hatred) would be too great. This means that the family environment is still the main educator for matters involving sexuality, gender, and violence. In previous chapters, I problematized the fact that the mother remains the most important family pillar for many communities in patriarchal societies (which still prevails on a global level). This means that a mother who has experienced any type of sexual violence – whether in war or not – will potentially present her at-home sexuality and gender education within this framework, at least to a certain extent. And if so many women deal with their own experiences of sexual violence though silence, we can only speculate about the sexual scripts, concepts, values, and patterns related to gender and sexuality that are transmitted at home, intentionally or not.

Literature in intergenerational research on the transmission of prejudices and intolerance at home shows that parents have a considerable impact on the broader value systems that model and contaminate children (for the literature review, see O'Bryan, Fishbein, & Ritchey 2004, 409). The findings of more recent studies indicate that intergroup attitudes develop as a result of bidirectional communication, where youth can also have an important impact on their parents or other adult authorities. An increasing amount of theoretical consideration is given to the tendency of youth to explore these issues themselves, and to "actively trigger responses from their parents, solicit parental behaviors, and influence their attitudes" (Miklikowska 2015, 5). When it comes to intolerance, the same sex-model based in psychoanalysis notes that girls resemble their mothers and boys their fathers in adopting prejudiced attitudes. O'Bryan, Fishbein, and Ritchey (2004, 410) mention the differential effects model, which furthermore assumes that mothers have different spheres of influence on the development of their children, depending on the children's sex and gender. Also mentioned is a study which found that the sexual attitudes of divorced mothers had an impact on their daughters but not their sons (in O'Bryan, Fishbein, & Ritchey 2004, ibid.). What these various studies agree on is the fact that young people generally feel closer to their mothers than to their fathers; they prefer to consult their mothers about their opinions and decisions, but also clash more often with their mothers.

As my interest lies beyond psychological processes, and I tend to focus more on community dynamics and the importance of group pressure on the individual, I find Carrie Paetcher's work on masculinities and femininities as *communities of practice* (2003) more helpful in developing an understanding of how and what aspects of toxic sexualities and gender relations might get transmitted from traumatized mothers (and fathers, too) in homes. For Paetcher, the process of learning masculinities and femininities happens in loose and overlapping communities of practice, where children and youth learn about and experience the expectations, behaviors, practices, and attitudes toward them as gendered individuals (Paetcher writes about male and/or female). According to her, a community of practice is therefore "a location in and through which individuals develop their identities, in relation both to other members of the community and to members of other communities" (Paetcher 2003, 7). She has developed her ideas based on Butler's premise that gender is performative (Butler 1993), but with the open question of *how one knows what to perform*, and how (if so) an individual's performance changes according to the circumstances.

Paetcher is furthermore skeptical that one can simply choose an identity, *to perform* anyone they want, arguing instead that identity is very intentionally learned and constructed through community induction and negotiation processes (Paetcher 2003, 152–155). This is why she also outlines possible intervention strategies to re-think and reconsider, as a community, whether we really want children still to identify as boys and girls as agreed within our communities of practice, or how to work on changing and adjusting these practices to the new orders. For an individual to remain a member of a particular community of practice, they must regulate, control, and adjust their performance to stay within the norms of that community – or find another one (Paetcher 2003, 15). If communities of femininity and masculinity practice therefore enforce what is perceived as the ideal, typical, desired version of female and male, how then can we understand how identity is constructed in communities where gender carries the burden of a never-resolved, violent past?

Identity as a learning trajectory is temporal, as argued by Wenger (1998, 55): in the process of negotiating the present, it incorporates the past and the future. But it is also locational, as argued by Paetcher (2003, 25): we take on and learn new and different identities every time we move from one place or institution to another. I would argue that the transition from war to postwar constitutes a change in place and institution that demands from the individual the construction of a new identity. Due to the complexity of identities and space prior to the war, and the many different experiences, cognitive self-explanations, and social agreements about war histories, it is an extremely hard task to identify and to maintain the complexity of these new postwar identities. However, I think here of the one collective identity that has been discussed a great deal among scholars of war-related rapes and sexual violence, and adopted and performed by many survivors – namely, collective victimhood.

Collective victimhood has become an orientation point for many survivors to find their place for their war experiences in postwar society. While it has become important to define the process, and it needs to be addressed during restorative justice processes, it is also helpful in collecting shattered traumatic memories into an understandable yet simplified narrative that allows many for personal healing and reintegration into society. For many survivors, the identity of war-rape victim and/or survivor has become central, yet at the same time inseparable from other identities such as gender, sexuality, ethnicity, nationality, and religion. As war rape is an attack on all those identities, the war-rape survivor in the aftermath of the war automatically reclaims all of them. As in any other identity construction, this reconstruction would necessarily involve "the Other," and this other is often also identified primarily by religion, ethnicity, and gender. Female war-rape survivors tend to be starkly distinct from other war survivors; hence, while ethnic and religious identity layers are important, what further separates survivors from society is how their gender and sexuality are to be reclaimed and reconstructed out of this very particular experience of abuse. This is also what distinguishes the mothering of these women from that of others, which makes sharing their stories with their children very often unimaginable.

To understand the identity construction of mother as it relates to the trauma of war rape, we might find a helpful example in Patricia Hill Collins's work, which takes *African American* mothering as a theoretical location that she believes "promises to shift our thinking about motherhood itself" (in Wenger 1998, 55). According to her, a *woman of color's mothering* consists of survival, identity, and empowerment. For these mothers, the physical (and psychological) survival of their children is central to their practices of mothering, as is everyday teaching about how to retain their identity in a dominant white culture, without becoming willing participants in their own subordination (Collins 1990, 123). Mother-work in a racially oppressive society means helping children to develop a meaningful racial identity within a society that continues to suppress this same identity – its history, culture, and belief systems. Unlike mothers from privileged social groups – in this case, white middle-class women – mothers of color must help their children to overcome regular negative representations, and to develop a mechanism to fight the inequality and discrimination that derive from this on an everyday basis.

A very similar intersection of survival, identity, and empowerment might be seen among war-rape survivors, though instead of focusing on the racial dimension (or any other identity labels, none of which are excluded), many survivors raise their girls and boys according to the patriarchally oppressive society in such a way that they can develop meaningful gender and sexual identities within a society that puts pressure on those same identities. This reflects back on the communities of practice mentioned above. In a context where mothers live in an oppressed community of practice, new members – children – learn to construct narratives of the self that accord with the mutual understandings of this very same community of practice; thus a shared pattern of personal and collective history is developed and supported (Paetcher 2007, 138). In order to break the cycles of oppression and to develop effective modes of resistance – against trauma transmission included! – Carrie Paetcher (2007, 155) suggests that we need to uncover the mechanisms of power structures in the construction of masculinities and femininities.

The limitation of these ideas lies in an empirical discrepancy: mothers do not necessarily teach resistance and empowerment because of their own personal experiences or because they mother in an oppressive context. As mentioned previously, I could note that mother–survivors strictly separate their survivor "activism" from their practices of mothering. I use the word "activism" here to refer to the (everyday) struggles of women involved in the processes of restorative justice: primarily survivors' sharing circles, but also including attending and contributing to juridical processes, and searching for and/or receiving reparations for physical and psychological harm. Some of the survivors actively participated in public events, commemorations, and media publications, but would never bring these topics into their homes. In many cases, the reason for this would be fear of transmission of trauma, and in others the potential for conveying (unintentionally) inflammatory, hateful, and divisive messages. One woman described her two roles as survivor and as mother, stating that she never plays these roles at the same time. "At home," she would say,

> I am a mother, and I want to be a role model for my daughter and for my son. I want my daughter to finish her schooling and be responsible. I want my son to be a good man, with respect. I want them to see my love for them, my tenderness and commitment. What happened to me during the war, this is my story and I share it here /sharing circle/, because other women here understand me. My kids, they cannot understand this, and they do not need to.
>
> (M47, Northern Bosnia 2018)

Survivors generally understand their survivor identity as something negative, a dark spot in their lives, but not necessarily as something that renders them powerless. On the contrary, as mothers, they "own" their identities, something that they like and of which they are proud. At home, they want to be mothers, but not necessarily also survivors. They want to be role models, and if asked if they feel responsible for how they raise their children, they would in most cases say yes. In this sense, motherhood is where they in fact place their agency; the home is a place where they feel they can teach, although not necessarily through direct sharing of their experiences or trauma. Instead, they stand for certain values (which are in most cases gender-based) and convey these to their daughters and sons. Gender-based values reflect nicely the ways in which violence was usually discussed with those who have sons. They felt responsible and emphasized the importance of teaching boys respect for women, not being violent, not drinking, and not leaving pregnant women alone. When it comes to the daughters, mothers mentioned values such as kindness, caring (especially for them when they get old), the desire to "give" them grandchildren, and finding a "nonaggressive" husband (from field work notes, July 2018, Northern Bosnia). My field work notes contain the following passage:

> While the identity of survivor is a consequence of a life event that they have not chosen on their own, and is an identity they would prefer not to have, but was in a way imposed on them, they feel that *the identity of the mother* is their calling, and so this is where it seems they want to place their agency. While they still feel powerless, disappointed and angry about the failures in the restorative justice process and the general attitude of state officials to the question of war-rape survivors, it feels that they held total control over the project of their mothering. It feels a place where they, too, can execute their power (not just being subjected to the use of power against themselves).
>
> (July 2018)

The agency of mothering also sometimes includes the desire for the repair of "historical failures": to raise their own children better than their parents and their grandparents raised them. In many cases they understand and recognize the femininities and masculinities communities of practices that allowed mass rapes to happen. Many would agree that mothers are to blame for their sons who rape; at the same time, they also feel a great responsibility not to be this kind of mother but, instead, a protector: to do everything to protect their children from the same or similar suffering. While these conversations tended to sound as though the women blamed their parents for not doing enough to prevent and/or stop the war, they also contradicted themselves later in the workshop. They spoke of how their mothers were "like angels" who were "always doing just the best for me," "she was pure gold," and "I know she would die just to protect me" (from field notes, July 2018). Placing the blame for past failures on an entire generation and reproaching "parents" for bequeathing a bad future to their children happened during one of the workshops I held with teenagers (June 2019). One boy explained that he feels annoyed that his generation has inherited such a "shitty state," having to deal now with a war that was not theirs.

I return to Patricia Hill Collins to reframe her concept of racial empowerment in terms of contextually more applicable ethnonationalistic politics: "we are standing still and proud for what /ethnic community/ was supposed to be gone by now, and disappear completely. But we are still here" (M46, Northern Bosnia 2019), says one survivor. An empowered daughter, as one interlocutor explained to me, is one who

> is not ashamed to cover, because today this is not seen as a virtue. I have never asked her to do this, but it makes me happy anyways. Because in her I can see that she got good values from me.
>
> (M46, Northern Bosnia 2019)

The relationship between empowerment through the practice of mothering as understood in Western feminist theory and empowerment as understood by the community of mother–survivors is complex. Survivors would call their practice empowered mothering because it is reflected through their own struggle of survival and postwar recovery. Confronting her violent past experience, and despite attempts to destroy her both physically and psychologically through the weapon of war rape, she mothers. Yet, in their practice of this view of empowerment, some mothers return to the values and social beliefs – the very system – that allowed the mass rapes to happen in the first place. I am not bringing this into the discussion to blame the mothers or to encourage the reader to assign guilt and responsibility for the perpetuation of intergenerational violence per se. But I will risk being misunderstood in attempting to develop an understanding of the impact and role of mothers entangled in complex, postconflict sociopolitical dynamics that are not only traumatizing, but which are also ideologically fueled and divisive, with governing bodies that promote radical identity politics and conflicting memory practices. The question of the responsibility of mothers was very often on the agenda of our meetings; however, those participating also almost always viewed "the other mothers" – not themselves – as being responsible for raising abusive children and/or nurturing hatred in their families. As for themselves, in most cases they conformed to the essentialist myths of innocence, kindness, and peacefulness. While I believe that socialization along the years involves different individuals, environments, and social groups, I also want to address with seriousness the issue of mothers' responsibility and reflect on how it could be better incorporated in existing peace education with youth. It is particularly important to note how (traumatized) mothers could generally undergo not only therapeutically oriented treatments to deal with their trauma, but also more socially oriented training to reflect on the role of mothers in the aftermath of conflict.

Understanding femininities and masculinities as communities of practice helps us to understand why traumatic sexual experiences stay with survivors and are easily transmitted to future generations. The notion of rape culture and the theoretical and empirical efforts to seize and deconstruct rape myths have been present in the social sciences since the introduction of second-wave feminism at the beginning of the 1970s. With the massive interest in the systemic, intentional, and planned use of rape as a weapon of war during the war in the former Yugoslavia in the 1990s, international law, academic communities, and the nongovernmental sector have succeeded in pushing forward several pivotal approaches to dealing with the recovery of survivors and their legacy in the community and on broader societal and political levels. Yet, the gendered and sexualized social configurations that allow and support the existence and cultural reproduction of rape culture are resistant to change. What is intriguing in the process of rape culture transference is not only how women (still) play a crucial role in it, but how war-rape survivors are sometimes incapable of understanding their own experience beyond their internalized, individualized, and privatized trauma.

In the traditional communities where most of my ethnographic research has taken place, children still perceive their parents – particularly their mothers – as powerful and significant members of their own community of practice. Thus, while survivors as mothers might engage with alternative ideas and lifestyles, concrete changes of their mothering practices are most likely to be slow; when they finally occur, they remain peripheral and unwanted. As mentioned previously, a mother will most likely feel she has failed if her children adopt values and patterns that differ from her own. Consequently, masculinity and femininity communities of practice, as fundamental constituents of one's identity, tend to maintain the status quo of traditional gender roles, divisions, and practices. This is most likely true even in situations where change is significant and where one would expect to see resistance to the "traditional" (Paetcher 2003, 26). I want to see a community of mothers who have survived war rape as a very particular femininity and masculinity community of practice, where engaging in a shared practice constitutes a mothering practice that is loaded with "tremendous social, cultural, political, economic, psychological and personal significance" (DiQuinzio 1999, viii).

The mothering of war-rape survivors is imbued with the experience of a profound trauma that assailed not only their own sexuality and gender. Forced impregnation was often part of intentional war rape policies, constituting an attack on women as potential mothers. War rapes that resulted in forced impregnation are therefore ideological and empirical sources of the female's most profound oppression, in which women "must suffer under the tyranny of nature, biology, and/or male control" (DiQuinzio 1999, ix). For some survivors, being attacked for the purpose of forced impregnation has forever changed not only their perspectives on motherhood but their practice of mothering. Through the forced impregnation of war rape, motherhood is radically essentialized. The ostensibly essential female characteristics of caretakers, such as the psychological and emotional capacity for empathy, recognition of the needs of others, and self-sacrifice were exploited to bring to life the perverse idea of the complete instrumentalization of women as individuals, transforming them into ethnicized wombs. Thus, the woman not only carries the baby of the perpetrator but delivers it and cares for its survival.

Motherhood in essentialist terms predicts that "all women want to be and should be mothers and clearly implies that women who do not manifest the qualities required by mothering and/or refuse mothering are deviant or deficient as women" (DiQuinzio 1999, xiii). In this way, the idea of forced impregnation depends on the cultural and social pressures that perceive maternity as natural to women and essential to their being: "they are born with a built-in set of capacities, dispositions, and desires to nurture children" (Courtenay Hall 1998, 59). Even forcefully impregnated women will therefore raise the child of the perpetrator, as her mothering instincts, dedication, and intuitive understanding surpass socially learned attitudes and skills. Forced impregnation policy – or impregnation for the purpose of genocide – is based on the belief that mothers will keep and raise these babies because they engage in loving them through unsocialized emotions (Courtenay Hall 1998, ibid.). While the patriarchal institution of motherhood is in any sense different from rape, prostitution, and slavery, all constrain, regulate, and dominate women (Rich in O'Reilly 2004, 33).

In *Of Woman Born*, a classic work on mothering and motherhood, author Adrienne Rich highlights two harmful characteristics of patriarchally regulated motherhood: in addition to "intensive mothering" (Hayes 1998), an assumption that child-rearing is natural to women and is thus the sole responsibility of the biological mother, this responsibility comes with no power to autonomously decide and determine how, in which way, to mother. Mothers are expected to mother by the rules defined by others; they do not create the rules but are expected to reinforce them. Motherhood, as explained by Rich, is an experience of "powerless responsibility" (in O'Reilly 2004, 6).

For this reason, feminist historians have developed counternarratives of motherhood to promote ways of mothering that empower women and which can be imagined and implemented outside of the patriarchal institution of motherhood. Andrea O'Reilly (2004, 10) introduces a new perspective that ascribes agency to mothers and defines mother-work as a socially engaged endeavor that

> seeks to effect cultural change in the home through feminist child rearing and the world at-large through political/social activism /.../ motherwork is…a socially engaged practice that seeks to effect cultural change through new feminist modes of socialization and interactions with daughters and sons.

DiQuinzio (1999, xv) similarly replaced the term "motherhood" with "mothering," not only to omit the ideological construct of essential motherhood but to emphasize maternal power in executing social change through a feminist rearing of boys and girls in the domain of the private sphere – the home.

Adrienne Rich, and the feminist scholars who have inherited her distinction between motherhood as an institution and mothering as a nonpatriarchal experience of children rearing, assumes that mothers recognize how performing traditional motherhood leads to traditional masculinity. That is, mothers who obtain power through mothering and the bond they have with their children are all oppressed and subjected to the father. For girls to grow into free, brave, and strong women, "we must be those women ourselves" (Arcana 1979, 33). Through mothering as a practice of agency, a mother models power and empowerment for the daughter, who will acquire those attitudes, self-sufficiency, and autonomy through the mother-daughter bond. At the same time, the practice of motherhood teaches daughters to "give in… that disastrously self-destructive way that has been honored by men as true motherhood," while the sons "learn to expect such treatment from women" (Arcana 1982, 102).

Feminist shift from an essentialist to a more poststructuralist understanding of motherhood can communicate several problematic notions when it acknowledges that empowered mothering would hardly come about without the influence of feminist thought. Various feminist theories and practices from the 1960s and 1970s viewed motherhood in a rather negative and simplistic way. According to Hester Einstein (1996, 69), the fact that "feminism and motherhood were in diametric opposition had seemed almost axiomatic in the early 1970s." This reminds me of feminist practice and the women-led antiwar movement in Yugoslavia, in which – as I mentioned earlier – women provided very few mother perspectives. This return to mothering, therefore, attempted to highlight the active nature of maternity as feminist thought sought to establish a space for women to reclaim the practice, separating it from patriarchal rule. However, the concept of mothering as developed by feminist mothers has claimed that agency would reflect general feminist aspirations. I could note that most of the mothers I have spoken to would agree on feminist agency and the struggles necessary to oppose patriarchally dictated subordination and the control of women and women's bodies. They would also see their own "agency," as mentioned above, in child-rearing, particularly in teaching their children to prevent and avoid traumatic experiences similar to what they have gone through. In some cases, the ways in which these mothers understand prevention should provoke some second thoughts about mothers – that is, survivors as potential accomplices in raising the next generation of perpetrators. Some survivors expressed that they experienced rape and abuse because men of their generation – brothers, fathers, husbands, partners – failed to protect them, or even more generally, failed to protect their land, their culture, their collective identity against the aggressor. "I am proud to say," says one of the women,

> that I have no more fear. I am proud to see my two sons, strong and with a lot of pride, I know they will always be there for me, I can always count on them.

They always worry about me, and I know they will be the first to protect me if something happens to me.

(Z48, Central Bosnia 2018)

Although I had a chance to meet one of her sons, unfortunately he did not respond to my invitation for a conversation. I would be eager to learn more about this mother-son relationship as well as the son's understanding of his own role. His mother told him about the rape. She told me that his reaction was anger, and

I better not tell him the name and last name and where he /her perpetrator/ lives, even though I know all this about him! I just know that S. /her son/ would go and kill him or just do something to him, or, God forbid, his family. Despite how much anger I feel, and sometimes I want to do the same, I don't want my son to do this – ever, God forbid! But it makes me feel good that he feels this way for me, I have to admit.

(Z48, Central Bosnia 2018)

Further conversations revealed that this survivor is not alone in her way of understanding the male protector role. There were others who believe, similarly, that it is the man in the family who must protect women, children, and the elderly. What was interesting, and this is perhaps the result of the communist legacy of an equal women workforce, survivors drew a distinction between economic and physical protection. While no one would say that the man must sustain them economically, they have seen biological, masculine strength as a means of protecting them; thus, though the man should be a protector, he is not necessarily a provider. The oppression of women in a patriarchal society should not therefore be seen as linear but always intersectional. To this end, it is also important to see the diverse levels of (dis)privilege that women enjoy in this oppressive intersectional relationship.

Even if mothering is a gendered activity, its hierarchical position differs greatly from mother to mother (Collins 1992, 95). For example, in almost every association where survivors gather in sharing circles, the equality and inclusiveness of all members is well represented on a discursive level and is a representational image of the group. On the other hand, it is clear that a survivor who represents the group usually possesses more capital, particularly social and symbolic, than its other members. These representatives have greater power when conducting outreach and participating in social and political activities related to restorative justice processes. Recently, the symbolic capital of these survivors has become very visible as recent public discourse on the survivors of rape has experienced some radical shifts. Lately, survivors are more often represented as strong heroines (though still with a victimhood identity), rather than the silent, forgotten, and abandoned victims of war. At the same time, there are those survivors who might follow the work of others but have never joined a group or spoken out about their own experiences. The reason for this often lies in other layers of their identities, such as class and/or economic dependency.

In this way, understanding empowered mothering is highly dependent on the sum of the (de)privileges of the individual survivors at the nexus of intersectional oppressions. And while many of the mothers I have been in contact with would value economic independence – among both daughters and sons – they would not necessarily reflect critically on other forms of patriarchal power. For instance, while they would encourage their daughters to study, receive a good education, and obtain a well-respected job, they would also express their expectation that their daughters become mothers. Like any other group identities, the "mother" identity comprises many components, some of which are highly contested. But what different variations of motherhood practices have in common is

> that they are dominated by stories clustering around the pressive forces that require the gestators and bearers of children – but not children's begetters – to keep children safe, tend to their physical needs, and teach the morals and manners that allow them to take their place in society.
>
> (Lineman Nelson 2001, 135)

To what extent can we therefore apply Rich's concept of mothering as a socially engaged enterprise that seeks to change gender socialization through new feminist modes when the stories clustered around mothers are mostly patriarchal? In Rich's thought, mothering tends to be perceived as an individual choice, and it is the mother's own decision to apply a feminist practice despite being immersed in a patriarchal context. When it comes to the restorative justice process, many survivors would perceive their struggle and their activism as feminist, and antipatriarchal, but this is not necessarily reflected in how they approach mothering. Sharing circles often allow survivors to exercise their feminist practice without unnecessary public exposure and without making themselves vulnerable in the context of their families and communities.

In the circle, mother-work becomes a shared practice and mothering an agency that can be appreciated, positively acknowledged, and respected by other survivors. But from this relatively safe bubble – where socially advanced practices are accepted – survivors return to households that in most cases remain patriarchally ordered and run. Among other things, sharing circles of survivors are also places of collective grief, where women can mourn their lost girlhood, recall the pre-abuse life, and exist in a space that welcomes and nurtures feminist thought. This is a place of empowerment, but very often with a clear boundary demarcating 'the bubble' from the outside world – the world of survivors' families. As mentioned earlier, the feminist thought in these circles is often limited to reflecting on the women's shared experience of war rape, but it also imposes social pressure in terms of executing traditional motherhood and the role of the mother in transmitting traditional, often conservative morals and values to their descendants.

This brings us back to Sara Ruddick's classic work on maternal thinking (1984) and a mother's *thought*: "the intellectual capacities she develops, the judgements she makes, the metaphysical attitude she assumes, the values she affirms" (Ruddick 1984, 214). Ruddick understands maternal thinking as reflective and intentional; the mother, in line with her own virtues, values, and beliefs, determines her mother-work and defines failure and success in her own practice of child-rearing. This arises from the social practices by which she is surrounded; namely, the ways in which people respond to social realities and the demands of those same realities. Ruddick believes that maternal practice always "responds to the historical reality of a biological child in a particular social world" (Ruddick 1984, ibid.). As women's premothering life experiences and opportunities vary greatly, so too will their ways of mothering. In a nationalistic and military context, women as (potential) mothers are granted the leading role in educating and encouraging children to live by the values prescribed in those contexts. To produce socially appreciable children, some women are led to embrace the culture of violence, exerting pressure on both daughters and sons to fulfill the values of the dominant culture.

Rather than speaking of the mother's actual adherence to the dominant rules and values, Ruddick speaks of conceptions of mothers' relations to those values. Raising an obedient child to fulfill these values is considered an achievement (Ruddick 1984, 221). Fearful of displeasing members of the dominant culture, a mother can find fulfillment among her own practice of mothers when her child is recognized as a full and respected member of this same culture (Ruddick, ibid.). It is important to read and re-contextualize Ruddick's work carefully to avoid blaming women or giving them full responsibility for child-rearing, even in patriarchal systems. The mother's role has always merged with the roles of other institutions, movements, and groups, and a woman who mothers is always helped, controlled, and/or navigated by other members of society who have an interest in shaping the growing child (see El-Bushra 2000; Afshar 2004). Nevertheless, says Ruddick (1984, 215), "a mother typically holds herself, and is held by others, responsible for the malfunction of the growth process." In societies across the globe and throughout history, most mothering practices happen in conditions where women possess little power and where, as they have to fulfill the values and desires demanded by others, their own values do not count. Acting against her own "authenticity" (Ruddick 1984, 221) and bearing the responsibility for the requests of others is a complete contradiction.

Under the concept of "powerless responsibility," Rich describes the conditions in which women are expected to mother in a patriarchal context where their agency is prescribed by others (in O'Reilly 2004, 7). This suggests a paradox of the practice of mothering, where women are required to undertake mother-work and are responsible (and blamed, if the child-rearing fails) to care for babies in accordance with the expectations of hegemonic norms patriarchal rules, values, and unequal gender power relationships. In Ruddick's theory of maternal work, a mother's responsibility lies in raising a child who will be socially accepted and feel a sense of belonging to their culture. O'Reilly, however, introduces the struggle of feminist mothers – who, I would claim, find themselves powerless – trapped in the absurd situation of allowing their children to grow up to become a part of their own social world, while at the same time resisting the rules and control of the larger patriarchal culture that constitutes this same world (O'Reilly 2004, 218).

In the controversial documentary film *The Red Pill* (2016), which explores the men's rights movement, Katherine Spillar, executive director of the Feminist Majority Foundation, claims that once a woman has been impregnated she "ultimately has the responsibility for this child." From the context of her talk and the work of her foundation, I believe that Spillar refers mostly to abortion rights. However, the controversies of woman's biological capacity to give birth, her own rights in deciding how to control this, and the responsibility put on her by a patriarchal society (especially if left alone with the child), should also ask to what extent mothers in such conditions therefore determine the continuity of generations. Whereas motherhood in a patriarchal society is controlled and directed by hegemonic patriarchal rule, child-rearing is women-centered – thus, children spend most of their time with their mothers, and "mothers are responsible for teaching children" (in Watson-Franke 2004, 80). Some scholars have shown an intensification of the conservative backlash, which has its roots primarily among adult survivors who attempt to reestablish the conditions for a "prewar" lifestyle. According to this mindset, young girls especially find themselves under the control of older generations (see for instance: Schnabel & Tabyshalieva 2012, 17).

Ruddick writes about the damaging social values and patterns that are perpetuated in patriarchal societies and how a "good" mother is responsible for endorsing these values for those in her care. As she is the person primarily responsible for raising children among socially respected individuals, this also means to train her

> daughters for powerlessness, her sons for war, and both for crippling work in dehumanizing factories, businesses, and processions. It may mean training both daughters and sons for defensive or arrogant power over others in sexual, economic, or political life.
>
> (Ruddick 1989, 221)

Thus, "powerless responsibility" implies that societies still hold mothers responsible for the (deviant) behavior of their children; yet they grant absolutely no power (of choice mostly) when deciding how to mother, which is usually precisely prescribed, specified, and directed.

When studying the behavior of postwar generations – the children and grandchildren of war-rape survivors – it is essential to situate that behavior within the context of significant family relationships; in the case of absent fathers, particularly the mother-daughter/mother-son dynamic. What behavioral attitudes reflect a sexually traumatized mother? Can a humiliated mother, encouraged by her own traumatic experience, turn toward the feminist practice of *mothering* while she lives and performs her mother-work in a context that recognizes any other practice but *motherhood* as her individual failure? Regardless of the oppressive patriarchal system, writes Fiona Joy Green (in O'Reilly 2004, 135), a feminist mother will explore the potential of overtly and covertly confronting oppressive power structures and the harm caused to individuals and collectives by social injustice produced through structural violence.

Furthermore, "the mother-daughter relationship is the ground for teaching, talking, and sharing the feminine experience and the more we empower that experience, the healthier our girls will be" (in Joy Green 2004, 163). When talking with survivors, I could align their thoughts with those of feminist scholars; however, the mothering practices of survivors are also infused with the fear and belief that their rape experiences are not exceptional, but rather cultural. This means that exposing their daughters to healthy feminist thought would essentially expose them as targets of (male) violence. Many maintain that obedience and silence are still the safest ways for women to survive the hazardous rules of their patriarchal surroundings, even though neither obedience nor silence helped to prevent the war's mass rapes.

> I always said to my T.: make yourself invisible in the street. Men are animals. But when you get your own man, when you marry, I promise you, you will rule his world. You will have your own place where you will be able to do whatever. But outside, don't provoke. They /men/ will use anything to go against you.
>
> (B64, Northern Bosnia 2018)

Many survivors have found strength and empowerment in the aftermath of war through child-rearing. But no matter how much their practice of mothering has been life affirming, the trauma involved in healing and in restorative justice agendas has been for many a completely separate yet simultaneous process. Although many have never shared their testimonies with their children, especially with their sons, they notice that their children have witnessed clues, and they fear that they have been humiliated through their experience and the healing process as well. In an interview with a mother and her daughter, the mother explained:

> Until I worked through my own self-hatred, and feeling humiliated after the war, I thought only of what she /her daughter/ sees. She sees me humiliated, powerless, I was dead and dysfunctional. I knew that I had to recover to be a role model and inspiration for her.
>
> (M52, Brčko 2019)

A mother–survivor who has experienced war rape does not, therefore, cope only with the existing patterns of a continuing oppressive system but must also incorporate the legacy of her mother's own traumatic past. Removing the burden of responsibility, I believe that the ethical social response is not only to provide psychotherapeutic support to help mothers heal from their trauma but it should extend further, particularly within institutional spaces of socialization. This includes, for instance, reconsidering how and in which way the traumatic legacy can be taught as a part of broader sex education both at home and in public institutions. It would be an important step in starting to address the transmission of trauma and, more concretely, toxic sexual scripts.

A survivor, a mother: The fear of fostering hatred

Despite reports from some survivors who claim that becoming a mother has helped them find a sense of purpose in the aftermath of war rape, the myth of motherhood that was perpetuated continuously throughout the war and despite changing circumstances also worked to cover up the psychological and physical damage endured by individuals and communities after the war. For many, protecting their children was an event more significant than the experience of rape. A survivor from central Bosnia-Herzegovina, for instance, told me that she was able to protect her two children while the rest of her family members vanished and have never been found. I can surmise from my many conversations with survivors that their priority has never been to acknowledge their own war experiences – to focus first on their own healing – but to either protect their already-born children or to become mothers and commit to mother-work after the war.

In many cases, when men vanished during the war, the mother was burdened with the responsibility of continuing to nurture not only her own children, but also other wounded or traumatized individuals. Mothering allows many survivors to harness the collective imagination of their role as peacebuilders, which manifests first through the sphere of their homes but is also believed to contribute to general social recovery (Schirch 2012, 64–65). It is methodologically challenging to consider the critical aspects of the theoretical paradigm while attempting to stay true to the nature of the field. It is as well challenging to avoid biological and essentialist paradigms of mothering, as well as the responsibility of women as mothers to transmit values, behavioral patterns, and – last but not least – trauma to their offspring, while the father is hardly noticed, mentioned, or acknowledged during my long-term ethnographic involvement. In this vein, ethnographic research with mother–survivors very often provides conflicting data to critical feminist thought that put so much effort in deconstructing the essentialist and naturalized understanding of women in peace and conflict.

Women's and mothers' involvement in peace movements and peacemaking has gone through its evolutionary stages, both in theory and empirically, and is of course contextual, spatial, and temporal. One of the major critiques is that, despite the perception of women as essentially peaceful – as opposed to essentially violent men – the role of women in the grandiose peacebuilding project, nationally and internationally, is assumed to be minor. But if one begins to perceive mothering as an initial peace education – including observing the power structures in the sphere of domestic life and the authoritative role of the mother in patriarchal societies – one might perhaps note that mothers can have a greater impact on sociopolitical life, sustainable peace, and postconflict recovery than one previously assumed. Or perhaps we do not want to see this domestic impact, since doing so would immediately result in reverting to the dangerous essentialism of the woman's role as mother. In societies that include a large number of absent fathers, is the impact of mothers not omnipresent in the grown adults who were raised by women? To seize upon this idea without risking essentialism or, worse, to point to mothers as being responsible for raising violent and abusive children, is a challenging task. I will anyway risk exploring further in this direction.

In 1991, at the beginning of the war in Yugoslavia, women were massively involved in antiwar protests; as noted by Cynthia Cockburn (1998, 38), "forty bus-loads of parents, mainly mothers, converged on the headquarters of the Yugoslav National Army, demanding the discharge of their sons." The first antiwar dem-onstrations in Serbia were initiated and led by women. When their sons were mobilized, mothers united and demanded that they be returned home; the antiwar peace caravan was also organized by a woman (Licht & Drakulić 1997; see also Popov-Momčinović 2013). Later, women were the first to engage in postconflict reconstruction and peacebuilding, but this can easily be backed up with argu-ments that do not base in any type of biological or natural explanations of peaceful 'nature' of women: men, many of whom are seriously wounded or simply vanish, are at the front, while those who remain – the women – care first for surviving family members, after which they are held responsible for the well-being of the broader community as well (Lich & Drakulić 1997).

While acknowledging the problematic archetype of woman as caretaker and the dangerous patriarchal definition of women's role in propagating nationalistic ideologies (see in Cockburn 1998, 38), I also want to note the immediate postcon-flict circumstances that have led many people, particularly women in rural areas, to return to the "known." After the chaotic and anarchist madness of the war, many survivors mentioned that they yearned for simple and predictable everyday situ-ations, relationships, and dynamics. Also, as much energy is needed for physical and mental recovery, complex sociopolitical schemes might be too demanding in the immediate aftermath of the war. When the war stops, life does not return to normal, because this normal has yet to be defined; the only normal at this point, therefore, consists of the known prewar culture and traditions – the daily routines that make them comfortable and with which they can still identify. I say "still" because sometimes identities during the war are so badly damaged that individuals need to reidentify themselves, a process that may involve reclaiming some of the old traditions, customs, and rituals. This is an interesting process of reintegration. While the war stripped many of their social roles, most of these people did not build new identities in the aftermath of the war but returned to what they were before – as though the war had been paused for a couple of years. I say it is interest-ing because war functions as a completely new social reality with its own rules and hierarchies, and many individuals acquire new identities – a guard, a detainee, a refugee, a witness, a victim – that are not analogous with any peacetime identities.

Despite the chaotic and anarchist nature of war, these new, afflicted identi-ties – the identity of war-rape victims, for instance – might be overwhelming and impossible to accept, as is postwar life in general. Thus, returning to the known, "the simple," "the predictable," is for many a natural response. From this perspec-tive, individuals who experience extreme sexual violence might not turn auto-matically against the oppressive patriarchal order that drives such violence. On the contrary, many would in fact continue to support it by accepting the shame, guilt, and other forms of submission that keep their rape experiences "theirs," private and intimate. War brings social change but does not disrupt established social patterns. War – and trauma in the aftermath of war – strengthens archaic identities and fosters the blossoming and perpetuation of "neo-traditional beliefs in a purported 'golden age' of patriarchal social rule" (Schnabel & Tabyshalieva 2012, 17) among new postwar generations.

An interesting manifestation of this "returning" to traditions that are not nec-essarily instilled by one's parents involves postwar trends in veiling practices among young Muslim women, for instance, particularly in Sarajevo. In a paral-lel study,[3] I led a conversation with a group of survivors and a group of covered Muslim girls in their 20s – that offered some inspiring introspection regarding the contradiction between the older generation's desired transmission of "traditional" and the "return to traditional" as taken over and appropriated by that generation's descendants. Whereas most of the survivors, despite their origins in rather rural areas, opposed the practice of veiling and viewed it is as peasant, archaic, and rural, my young interlocutors saw it as a matter of personal choice and pride. For the survivors, the covering of women arose from the demands of patriarchal rule, and they believed their grandmothers fought for the free choice to cover:

> Our mothers were good Muslims, but they wear *dimije* and scarf, of course. But she understood that I was young and that I wanted to be like the others. She told me she would like me to wear *dimije*, but she never forced me. I wear jeans, you know! If these women want to be traditional, if they want to be real Bosniaks, they could wear *dimije*, but they wear jeans too and then they a put scarf over their heads. Tell me how this goes together!
>
> (S49, Sarajevo 2018)

Another survivor mentioned several times how women's dress has been discussed throughout history and how it is related to their honor and "purity." However, such control and social "protection" has not prevented women from being sexu-ally violated or raped:

> It never does. Women were never safe, no matter if they covered or not. They are telling us to cover, to take care of our attitudes and how we behave. But in the end, you are a victim anyway. I behaved well, but they raped me.
>
> (K57, Sarajevo 2018)

Another survivor explained that, in her opinion, reveiling represented the indi-vidual's or community's renegotiation of the war's attempted ethnic cleansing, revealing an urge to somehow manifest Muslim culture physically in postwar Bosnia-Herzegovina. She continued, noting that veiling today connects what "has been left" and what "remains of us," even if "we don't even think about the fact that the veil was once brought to the Balkans and was new to women at one point in history." She herself argued that although she barely wore a veil before the war, she started to use it in the aftermaths as it helps her to "find a connection to the life before the war" (S49, Sarajevo 2018).

Women who survived rape during the war see their roles as mothers as being of great importance, especially when it comes to teaching their offspring – particularly girls – about the dangers of their patriarchal surroundings. While most of the survivors believe that they must teach their daughters to cook and care for those around them – in short, to become good mothers – they also believe that veiling is an old tradition that is today rather imposed and unnecessary. In contrast, the group of young Muslim women in that research expressed their view that veiling is not imposed by anyone but is their own decision, as any other like education or being financially independent. They did not see religion and education as exclusive, nor did they view religion and the traditional dress that has its roots in religion as archaic, or "not ours" While for the survivors veiling was part of the "old times," the group of young women would not even perceive it as a "traditional."

The veiling practices of young Muslim women in today's Bosnia are very complex and nuanced, and I do not want to draw any simplistic conclusions, as doing so would require a more specific focus. However, I wanted to bring in this example because it is related to women's bodies in public and private spaces, and sexuality, and because it simultaneously shatters some of our stereotypical ideas about how we understand "traditional," how women can support patriarchy, how certain practices can be contradictory, and particularly how traditions are not simply transmitted to succeeding generations but are also actively (though perhaps critically) adopted, readjusted, and changed by new generations. I offered this example to remind us also that, no matter what mothers aspire to teach their children, those children will find inspiration elsewhere. This is particularly important when we consider the impacts of mothers' traumas, and responsibility of mothers in teaching peace (or hatred).

Women in the aftermath of war may also draw on traditional gender roles and identities for other, more pragmatic reasons. Being occupied with looking after children, rebuilding homes, and managing the house not only allows them to reestablish and normalize life after the disaster, but also demonstrates some healing effects in coping with trauma. For many of my interlocuters, children symbolized hope and life, and also made them determined not to give up on their own lives, despite everything they had survived and witnessed (see also the comparative example of Mozambican women in Sideris 2001, 152). While warfare operates through traditional patriarchal divisions, leaving villages and other places to be run by those who have not vanished – very often women and children – the burden of caring for children and the elderly often rests increasingly on the shoulders of women (Danopoulos, Skandalis, & Isakovic 2012, 145). Thus, the impact of war on gender roles and family dynamics can be seen as the logical outcome of how war is waged. Krishna Kumar has noticed how the workload for women in Bosnia-Herzegovina increased dramatically in the aftermath of the war,

> as they have to assume greater economic and social responsibilities in view of growing poverty and hardships. … they have to continue to perform tasks

such as cooking, washing clothes, and caring for children, as well as spending more hours on farm work or other jobs.

(Kumar 2012, 84)

Despite valuable feminist writings on the need to deconstruct essentialist and biologized ideas of women in the fight against patriarchy, most survivors needed to react and respond immediately, leaving them with little choice to consider and exercise alternative, nonessentialist mothering. Mothering and caregiving appears *natural* due to women's innately peaceful essence, but is instead a result of the logistical organization of war, in which men, many of whom have vanished, are mostly absent. When fearing the reproduction of essentialist thought, one must also be realistic and consider the conditions and resources with which mothers were equipped when confronted with a postwar life. The ethnographic data show that the gap between theory and praxis is nevertheless present. For example, many of my interlocutors would like to see themselves as nurturing, emphatic, supportive, and emotionally sensitive to others. Very often, her experience of violence would be presented as an incentive that induces her to teach her children in such a way that would prevent these dreadful things from ever happening again, to anyone. When teaching peace or hate, most would see their homes as the primary place where peace education starts. But how is *peace* defined among the mother–survivors?

In an unstable postconflict country such as Bosnia-Herzegovina, peace is not simply the absence of direct violence, especially not for women (Bailey 1992, 101). In terms of armed conflict, there has been no direct violence in the country since the Dayton agreement of 1995. However, other types of violence – discursive, political, symbolic, and structural – present continuous stress that causes people to be alert and prepared to triggers that have the potential to significantly affect family life. For many survivors of rapes and sexual violence, the path to peace correlates with the cases of other war victims that are involved in restorative justice processes and with a general peacebuilding plan that is part of a broader (inter)national project. As I tried to explain in the previous chapter, survivors follow this process at very different levels of their "silence": some are very active and engaged, some are observers, and some are trying only to get over it, dealing only with the challenges of their everyday life as though the war had never happened. I have been discussing with survivors their own perceptions or definitions of peace and how they as individuals practice peacebuilding as a bottom-up process. I suggest locating their answers in one of three nonhierarchical levels:

1. *Inner individual peace*: coming to terms with the violent past; understanding what happened in a cognitive and emotional way; working through the pain; finding her own ways of communicating the traumatic events within her family and with the broader society; or alternatively, finding her own path to mental and physical recovery, no matter if the surrounding environment accepts or rejects her.
2. *Peace inside her family and extended family*: having been accepted, having a space to safely share her experience and its traumatic legacy; having support

from family members; feeling safe and welcomed enough to share her emotions related to triggers or PTSD.

3. *Achieving peace in society*: the state's response to her needs as a survivor; her story being heard and acknowledged; her rights related to financial and medical needs that must be met; society shifting the blame from the survivors to the perpetrators; war rape stories as part of cultural memory, with the important political representatives joining the commemorations.

These levels are not hierarchical because one level does not need to be attained in order to move on to the next one; they are also not in any presupposed order. One survivor told me about her supportive family environment and especially the great support she receives from her daughters; even so, she said, her struggles to achieve inner peace and to come to terms with the past in her own psychotherapeutic work would continue despite this support. In another, similar experience, a survivor who gave birth to the child of rape continues to blame herself for not leaving the country before the war started, even though her son has dealt positively with their story and remains by her side. In another, different story, a survivor finds her "peace" among other women, but never in her family; when meeting with other survivors, she feels she can be who she is; she feels she has no fear but only hope that her life will again come together. Her anxiety starts again as soon as she finds herself on the streets and returns home from the space that she considers 'safe': sharing circles of other survivors, social centers, and associations that offer support and different activities for the survivors.

Similar to the very diverse mechanisms used to cope with the silence, survivors also have extremely diverse ways of recovering and achieving peace at those different levels. What effect does this peace journey have on their mothering? How is their own state of peace – inner, individual, or social – conditioned by the transmission of their traumas and potential hatred of their offspring? The essential demands placed on a mother in fostering growth and preserving love ignore the struggles she experiences in meeting her own survival needs, such as loving care, protection, tenderness, and healing. The essentialism of a universal mothers' love assumes that those deprived of love, first as daughters and later as women exposed to the radical violence of war, nevertheless find within themselves the resources to *nurture* others – that is, within this ostensibly biologically predisposed tendency. In this essentialist version of a mother's love, the woman herself does not need to be loved and nurtured but will be expected to give love if she is to become a mother.

Due to the suffering caused mainly by PTSD, many who care for and love their children expend a great deal of emotional energy that is only rarely recognized. Mothers who find themselves unable to love their children unconditionally or who focus on their own psychological recovery and traumatic legacies are often faced with feelings of inadequacy, blame, and guilt. The biggest failure for survivors is not their inability to recover and heal from their own trauma, but their inability to love their children unconditionally because of that same trauma. In cases where their children are not fully adjusted to their social surroundings, they are furthermore "second guessed by legions of self-proclaimed experts, other family members" (Edmonds 2009, 206).

On a daily basis, mother–survivors must find ways to integrate their own traumatic experiences – which symbolize *regression* in their own, individual, personal development – with the *progressive* attitude of fostering care and love despite having been subjected to extreme violence, abandonment, and hatred. Furthermore, survivors must "foster stability within the context of change; protect without thwarting autonomy; and exert control when they possess relatively little power themselves" (Edmonds 2009, 205). Navigating mother-work in this demanding and complex social sphere in the aftermath of war, while simultaneously trying to manage her own symptoms of posttraumatic stress disorder, is extremely challenging. Yet this work never receives any public recognition or awards. The only peacebuilding activity per se is to glue back together the pieces of shattered societies and attempt to normalize life in the aftermath of the war.

However, what might be understood as loving and nurturing within protective dimensions might edge very closely to the narrative which states that the "Other" is rather untrustworthy and best avoided. At this point, loving and protecting her own child might instead communicate distance and avoidance of the "other" child. For this reason, most survivors – for reasons due primarily to fears of another, new conflict in the name of children and family – prefer their children to live in monoethnic and monoreligious environments (see also: Schirch 2012, 21). This should not automatically imply prejudice or hatred; rather, survivors often feel that they lack the necessary communication skills and social competencies to reestablish interethnic relationships following the atrocities. This occurs in contexts where most communities are systematically and institutionally divided, and where the system is organized in such a way that there is no need to collaborate or establish contact with the "other side." To prove their openness and tolerance, mothers would often tell me that they had girlfriends from all ethnic groups before the war and that they have maintained these relationships. However, to foster intergroup trust, tolerance, and collaboration in a society that was affected so badly – as in the case of the Bosnian war – it is very hard to draw any conclusions, especially when one's only connection to the other side is a prewar friend who vanished, or a perpetrator living in the neighborhood who has never been brought to justice and continues to enjoy a respected position in the community.

The relationship with "the Other" is therefore a more or less principled attitude and has little in common with the concrete practices of coexistence. After I finished a meeting with a survivor, her son picked us up in order to drive me to the bus station. We stopped along the way for the mother to pick up some things in a kiosk, which gave me the chance to briefly engage in conversation with her son. He told me:

> Until the end of primary school I was not even aware that there are "different" people, if you know what I mean. Only when I had to transit to another town to start secondary school, I realized that we can be identified by different names, and this was when I became interested in what happened here during

the war. I don't think I have ever selected my friends on the basis of their ethnic affiliation, but I do remember that I was confused at first.

(R26, Central Bosnia 2018)

When I later met his mother alone at some other occasion, I asked her if she had ever talked with her son about the country's postwar ethnic divisions, to which she responded:

> I did not. But not because I would have some type of hatred toward /ethnic group omitted/. But honestly, let me tell you, I was afraid if I would tell him, that he would hate them. And I don't want him to hate anyone. I want him to have friends among /ethnic group omitted/ even though I must say that I always fear. I also fear that they would tell him lies.
>
> (S48, Central Bosnia 2019)

Mother–survivors I've spoken with often feel proud to be called upon – as though it were their duty – to nurture peace and prevent future violence. When I asked them if they "teach peace," one group always confidently confirmed that, despite what happened to them, they would never fuel their children with hatred and prejudice toward another ethnic group. Another group said the same, adding that they do not "really encourage my daughter to meet with the other side – not because I hate them, but because I do not totally trust them." (R41, Mostar 2018). At a summer school in Mostar in 2018, a boy in my class shared how his mother was always hesitant to let him cross a certain bridge because "the kids there will bully you" (from fieldnotes, July 2018). In another example, a survivor shared her fears:

> I have never raised my kid with hatred toward the other. But some mothers are like this. I know my girl was bullied in school from a /ethnic identity/ boy. Namely, his mother tells him to hate us. I just want to protect my girl, and I am happy that she will now go to the secondary school in /town name/.
>
> (Z47, North-East Bosnia 2018)

The "otherness" that supports existing divisions and which somehow plays against reconciliation is therefore conveyed through the apparently positive process of protection. This draws interesting parallels with the general war discourse, in which war crimes are justified through the ideas of protection and resilience. In conversation, survivors stated explicitly that they do not promote hatred toward the "Other." Most do not lead any conversation with their children at all, thus dealing with their own symptoms and recovery process in silence. When they do share, they claim to "warn" the children to be careful with the "Other," arguing mostly that this is a good faith caution to protect them from bullying, hatred, and exclusion:

> I did not raise my son to kill others, but to protect me and our family. We were targeted and killed while innocent and unarmed. I do not want my son to do this. But if someone comes and attacks me, I want him to protect me.
>
> (M67, Sarajevo 2018)

When I asked this group of women if they believed that the "protection" narrative might in any way backfire or prevent reconciliation among the divided populations, one of the survivors answered:

> I did not forget what these people did to me. This means they were raised in this manner. Someone raised a man to rape, am I right? Why would I now believe that they have changed? Not all, I am not saying all are the same. But they have this now in the history. They can raise a rapist. And of course I am thinking of my daughter, being together with /ethnic identity/ boy in the school, and yes, I will tell you, I think he is capable of doing the same as their men did in the war to me. Of course I want to protect her, I don't say to hate their boys, I say – be careful!
>
> (R, Sarajevo 2018)

What is the notion of protection in war and where are the limitations of such discourse? Isn't war always *protecting* – that is, killing before we can get killed, raping before we get raped, expelling before we get expelled? What, therefore, is the relationship between nurturing intercultural hatred and protecting "our" values, "our" territories, and "our" people?

Hatred, according to psychoanalytic theories, develops as a means of protecting an infant from threats, mainly pain and danger; it is one of the most basic survival strategies. In adulthood, hatred remains the same defensive mechanism except that it now protects one from social (economic, political, and other) conditions that are, or appear to be, threatening (see Klein 1962; also: Blee 2004). Postconflict hatred is a much more nuanced response that includes social and personal instability, inherited fears, and last but not least, symptoms of PTSD. Rooting hate in psychosocial analysis, therefore, risks limiting our understanding of a phenomenon that has broader social implications, especially when it comes to the collective hatred one group has for another group and when this collective hatred traces a long history of unresolved, disputed, and politically manipulated relationships (Ahmed 2004; Zembylas 2007).

However, it is challenging to draw conclusions from ethnographic evidence which suggests that survivors can be as openly hateful of and hostile toward the "Other" as the perpetrator's group. This is due partly to the inefficiency of methodological approaches that allow individuals to overcome their moral positioning and explore their own emotions in the very process of the research. I am always combining traditional ethnographic methods based on language expression with alternative, more ad hoc methods, which could help to position the tendency to protect within the frame of potentially hate-inducing patterns. A powerful experience that helped me to grasp the questions related to hatred and vengeance among survivors was an act performed in one of the workshops in 2013, during which several survivors expressed the need for a space where they could vent their negative and destructive emotions. After the activity, some of the women explained that, having vented their anger and frustration with failed justice procedures, they would no longer desire to get real-life revenge on their rapist/perpetrator, even if the circumstances would allow it. When asked to stage a scenario in which they meet their perpetrator and engage in some encounter with them, two of the women commented:

> I wanted to use this chance because you said one of us will play the man. I know I am full of hate, but I know it's not nice. I will be happy, yes, I will be very happy, if this man who did this to me goes to court and yes, I want to see him on TV and in jail. Maybe I want to kill him, but what then – I will only be like him. And I know I am better. But when you said, we can just act this out as a play, I wanted to try what I feel.
>
> (M, Central Bosnia 2013)

> When you asked /name omitted/ to go and meet her rapist, I felt anxious but also somehow excited. I want to tell this man a lot of things. I want to tell him what he did to me. Maybe I want to kill him if you give me the chance. But I think it's not good. It will just make me as bad a person as they are. If I know we are here, hidden, I want to feel how it feels if I know I can kill him. But if you want to write this now for the newspaper or your book, you shouldn't write this about us.
>
> (S, Central Bosnia 2013)

One of the women expressed that she understands that (physical) revenge, such as murder or/and threats, is not the answer and that if victims do seek or overtly desire revenge, then this "war will never stop." She explains:

> I know, maybe I want to kill this man. Yes, if I meet him again, I would attack him, this is how full of hate I am. But now I am a mother. I know I can't tell this to my daughter. Maybe she will think I am serious. Maybe she will want to kill this man. Hence, this will never stop.
>
> (A, Central Bosnia 2013)

This woman did acknowledge the importance of and the need for forgiveness in order to build a postwar life and postwar society. She feels that, without forgiveness, hatred, the desire for vengeance, and – in the worst cases – cycles of revenge and counter-revenge will not end. I will elaborate on the interconnectedness of these emotions in the next book section. For now, it is important to return to how women "warn" their children to be careful with the "Other" side:

> I can't forget and I will never be able to forget what has been done to us. But I don't want my daughter to be affected by this. What has been done has been done. If she hates them /she refers to another ethnic group/ I will become like them, and they only know how to hate. And I think we can't forgive, because we don't think hate is good. But we need to live. But I can't forgive.
>
> (A, Central Bosnia 2013)

While the above cases illustrate how survivors feel anger and hate toward the perpetrators, they also illuminate the survivors' feelings of frustration over an ineffective and slow justice system that allows the great majority of these perpetrators to remain free and lead completely normal lives. These kinds of embodied work also show that most survivors do not morally accept emotions such as hate and vengeance, so they intentionally suppress them to prevent their being transferred to the next generation.

While a strong victimhood identity often establishes the illusion that the victim is essentially "better" than the perpetrator – hence the strong stance against hatred to mask anxiety or any parallels with the perpetrator – I find it more useful to refer to the concept of the "pedagogy of suffering" elaborated by Frank W. Arthur (2003) when trying to understand survivors' emotional attitudes toward the other side (the perpetrator as a collective). Arthur uses the term to describe the wounded storyteller – the ill person and what they can teach society through their own experience of battling the disease. Of course, viewing rape survivors as ill people would not only be epistemologically misleading, but also morally wrong. Rather, the very act of rape and the sociopolitical approach toward dealing with its consequences is a *historical social disease* inflicted on communities, particularly women. The pedagogy of suffering, claims Arthur, calls for listening to the one who suffers, as she has "something to teach ... and thus ... has something to give" (2003, 150). While most survivors find it incredibly important to have a space to share their trauma stories, for many it would be ideal if those stories could also be heard by their descendants.

But these same stories can in fact teach fear, hate, and mistrust (Ramanathapillai 2006; Kinnvall 2013). To overcome the negative emotions involved with trauma stories – particularly vengeance and hatred – Zembylas emphasized the importance of developing empathy and returning humanity toward the Other (Zembylas 2007a, 207). The process of rehumanization (Halpern & Weinstein 2004) is not to internalize the emotions of the other, but to see that person in human terms – imagining the "enemy" from a particular perspective that draws on commonalities, or "How is 'the Other' similar to me?" Like hatred, empathy might appear too conceptual to many, and one can find it particularly difficult to apply in a context that involves an extremely unbalanced power relationship; where several state political bodies collaborate to cover up the crimes; where victims and survivors who obtain sufficient evidence and testimonies to bring the case to legal prosecution are instead laughed at, shamed, and sometimes threatened; and, finally, where the very crime of rape has no real mitigating explanations that survivors could use in their efforts to rehumanize the perpetrator and to reduce the moral or legal culpability of the guilty individuals and collectives. There are questions that arise when empathy is discussed in the context of forgiveness, reconciliation, and moving on, in which it is not always possible – cognitively, emotionally, and morally – to imagine the perspective of the Other within the perpetrator-victim relationship.

As in any other situation, it is unfair to generalize and homogenize either the perpetrator's or the victim's experiences, role, social status before/during/after the war, and the very circumstances and conditions in which crimes have been committed. While we must take into consideration the men who were forcefully mobilized and forced to commit rapes – putting them in the position of captives, as with any other victim – there were also those who accepted the chaotic and anarchic "rules" of war, those who enjoyed exercising their newly obtained powers and dominance, in which "imagining the particular perspective of the Other – that is, realizing that the Other is like me" (Zembylas 2007, 208), could very easily communicate controversial messages. In the context of the Bosnian war, we witness the persistent lack of data about 'the Other' side – particularly testimonies and evidence from the side of the perpetrators that might help us to understand fully the meaning of the crimes committed and the responsibilities for which individuals and communities should be held to account. After leading a long and nuanced conversation with a group of women in Northern Bosnia in September 2018, I wrote in my diary:

I don't even feel myself that empathy is something to be nurtured with the belief that it will prevent negative and destructive emotions from being transferred to the next generation. If I only imagine a woman sending her daughter to a school where she is continuously bullied and sexually harassed, and the only response would be to teach the daughter empathy and understanding toward the bully boy, what messages do we convey in terms of structural violence (in this case gender-based/sexual violence)? There must be punishment before empathy. There must be regret before empathy. It seems that the general psychosocial support that women are receiving would also have to include a guided process of dealing with the so-called destructive emotions, like hate. I could see that only when I acknowledge that perhaps hate is not a "wrong" emotion would they open up a bit more and share – in fact, their fears for the hate they feel. It was also evident that they are aware that hate will not lead them anywhere. But does this mean that we should completely ignore it in psychotherapeutic practice with survivors?

I thus find it extremely difficult to identify a place for empathy in the psychosocial recovery of survivors and feel hesitant about applying it in peace education programs. Cultivating empathy furthermore demands some type of encounter between the parties to be reconciled. For most survivors, this means a distant encounter in the official setting of a court procedure; for some, it would mean following the occasional news item concerning the prosecution process; for others, in cases where the perpetrator lives in the same area as the survivor, it would mean random meetings on the street or at public services. As there is no dialogue and no formal or informal platform for the parties in conflict to meet, individuals may generate a rather artificial and abstract emotional relationship toward the perpetrator.

Sometimes, loss – including the experience of war rape, but also other war-related losses such as vanished family members, burnt property, postwar humiliation, and revictimization – is so painful that brutalizing and dehumanizing the perpetrator is the only way individuals might cognitively and rationally comprehend the crimes committed. Therefore, the role of empathy might apply in the context of education and with the survivor's descendants, in which a particular individual carries the collective identity of the victims/survivors as well as the responsibilities that come with it. But in the context of the current sociopolitical situation in postwar Bosnia-Herzegovina, thinking of empathy is not just utopic, it also disregards many of the survivors' efforts and demands involving the restorative justice process.

I want to look at a very concrete example as a way to think about and understand other emotional tools that mother–survivors can use to avoid the negative emotions that derive from their traumatic experiences and subsequent posttraumatic stress symptoms. Most mother–survivors would agree that hatred must be overcome, and that reconciliation at some point is needed, and that they aspire to have their children live in a reunited community and be loving and caring being – to everyone, despite their ethno-religious, racial or gendered identity. For these same reasons, many hesitate to share their testimonies or perspectives on war events with their children out of fear that their children would be unable to distinguish between the act of the perpetrator and their crime, and the burdensome legacy that the community from the "other side" must carry in the aftermath of the war. Survivors openly express that it would be only natural for their children to react angrily and in a defensive and protective way toward their mothers; that rage, hatred, and in some cases vengeance would be a very natural and somehow predictable reaction. To prevent this, many decide to keep silent, using their sharing circles as a place of their "past" and their families as their "future."

Most of the mother–survivors with whom I have engaged in conversation, therefore, see themselves as peace educators and peace promoters at home. However, even if never explicitly stated aloud, there has always been this imaginary other, *the bad mother*, who is not among "us" and is very different from "us." This is, in fact, the mother who raises a perpetrator, the mother who has raised the men who became rapists. This mother, although abstract and nameless, is pointed at without any mother-to-mother solidarity. While mothers confirmed to me throughout our conversations that mothers are to be accused and held responsible for raising perpetrators, they also confirmed the myth of the *good-peaceful-and-nurturing-mother-only* when asking me very loudly, "But what kind of woman would teach her son to rape?" (M62, Central Bosnia 2019).

Notes

1 Generally, scholars of the Srebrenica massacre omit the term "gendercide" because using it may seem to belittle the genocide committed in Bosnia-Herzegovina. However, the use of the term gendercide in the context of this text seems important because it emphasizes how, after the mass murder of men and boys, female-headed households

became a reality for almost 40 percent of the internally displaced people who escaped from Srebrenica (in Simić 2009, 224). Because of this, women from traditional house-holds were challenged to examine their social/gender roles and the notion of traditional motherhood (Simić 2009).

2 The link to the conference report is not active (attempt to access: 8 August 2018).

3 See Močnik, Nena (2019). "Occupying the land, grabbing the body: The female body as a disposable place of colonialization in post-Ottoman Bosnia-Herzegovina." *Southern Europe* 43: 93–110.

Bibliography

Åhäll, L. 2012. "Motherhood, myth and gendered agency in political violence." *International Feminist Journal of Politics* 14 (1): 103–120.

Ahmed, S. 2004. *The cultural politics of emotions*. Edinburgh: Edinburgh University Press.

Ahmetasevic, N. 2010. *Women victims of sexual abuse in the Srebrenica genocide*. Available at https://www.scribd.com/document/34161869/Women-Victims-of-Sexual-Abuse-in-the-Srebrenica-Genocide (accessed 8 August 2018).

Ahrens, C. E. 2006. "Being silenced: The impact of negative social reactions on the disclosure of rape." *American Journal of Community Psychology* 38 (3–4): 263–274.

Albanese, P. 2001. "Nationalism, war, and archaization of gender relations in the Balkans." *Violence against Women* 7 (9): 999–1023.

Allen, B. 1996. *Rape warfare: The hidden genocide in Bosnia-Herzegovina and Croatia*. Minneapolis: University of Minnesota Press.

Arcana, J. 1983. *Every mother's son: The role of mothers in the making of men*. New York: Anchor Press.

Asfar, H. 2004. "Introduction: War and peace: What do women contribute." In H. Afshar and E. Deborah (Eds.), *Development, women and war: Feminist perspectives* (1–10). Oxford: Oxfam.

Bailey, A. 1996. "Mothering, diversity, and peace: Comments on Sara Ruddick's feminist maternal peace politics." In K. J. Warren and D. L. Cady, (Eds.), *Bringing peace home* (88–105). Bloomington: Indiana University Press.

Blee, K. 2004. "Positioning hate." *Journal of Hate Studies* 3 (1): 95–106.

Bolkovac, K. and Lynn, C. 2011. *The whistleblower: Sex trafficking, military contractors, and one woman's fight for justice*. New York: Palgrave Macmillan.

Bowcott, O. 2005. *Report reveals shame of UN peacekeepers: Sexual abuse by soldiers 'must be punished*. Available at https://www.theguardian.com/world/2005/mar/25/unitednations (accessed August 9, 2018).

Bracewell, W. 1996. "Women, motherhood, and contemporary Serbian nationalism." *Women's Studies International Forum* 19 (1–2): 25–33.

Burchianti, M. E. 2004. "Building bridges of memory: The mothers of the Plaza de Mayo and the cultural politics of maternal memories." *History and Anthropology* 15 (2): 133–150.

Butler, J. 1993. *Bodies that matter: On the discursive limits of "sex."*. New York: Routledge.

Chodorow, N. 1978. *The reproduction of mothering: Psychoanalysis and the sociology of gender*. Berkeley: University of California Press.

Cockburn, C. 1998. *The space between us: Negotiating gender and national identities in conflict*. New York: Zed Books.

Cockburn, C. 2004. "The continuum of violence: A gender perspective on war and peace." In W. Giles and J. Hyndman (Eds.), *Sites of violence: Gender and conflict zones* (24–44). Oakland: University of California Press.

Cogan, K. 2013. "The stitching mothers of Srebrenica v. Netherlands." *American Society of International Law* 104 (4): 884–890.

Collins, P. 1992. "Shifting the centre: Race, class and feminist theorizing about motherhood." In D. Bassin (Ed.), *Representations and motherhood* (371–388). New Haven: Yale University Press.

Copelon, R. 1995. "Gendered war crimes: Reconceptualizing rape in time of war." In: J. Peters and A. Wolper (Eds.), *Women's rights, human rights: International feminist perspectives* (197–214). New York: Routledge.

Danopoulos, C., Skandalis, K., and Isakovic, Z. 2012. "Women and children in the post-cold war Balkans: Concerns and responses." In A. Schnabel and A. Tabyshalieva (Eds.), *Defying victimhood: Women and post-conflict peacebuilding* (145–165). New York: United Nations.

DiQuinzio, P. 1999. *The impossibility of motherhood: Feminism, individualism and the problem of mothering.* New York: Routledge.

Djurić-Kuzmanović, T., Drezgić, R., and Žarkov, D. 2008. "Gendered war, gendered peace: Violent conflicts in the Balkans and their consequences." In D. Pankhurst (Ed.), *Gendered peace: Women's struggles for post-war justice and reconciliation* (265–291). New York: Routledge.

Duhan Kaplan, L. 1994. "Woman as caretakers: An archetype that supports patriarchal militarism." In Karen J. Warren and Duane L. Cady (Eds.), *Bringing peace home: Feminism, violence, and nature* (165–174). Bloomington: Indiana University Press.

Edmonds, R. 2009. "Maternal thinking expanded: A psychologist's view." In A. O'Reilly (Ed.), *Maternal thinking: Philosophy, politics, practice* (204–216). Toronto: Demeter Press.

Einstein, Z. 1996. *Hatreds: Racialized and sexualized conflicts in the 21st century.* New York: Routledge.

El-Bushra, J. 2000. "Transforming conflict: Some thoughts on a gendered understanding of conflict processes." In S. Jacobs, R. Jacobson, and J. Marchbank (Eds.), *States of conflict: Gender, violence and resistance* (66–86). London: Zed Books.

Frank, W. A. 2003. *The wounded storyteller: Body, illness and ethics.* Chicago: University of Chicago Press.

Gallimore, R. 2017. "Genocide and the killing of motherhood, mothering and maternal body: Their rehabilitation in post-genocide Rwandan society." *The International Journal of Conflict & Reconciliation* 3 (1): 1–35.

Hall, P. C. 1998. "Mothering mythology in the late 20th century: Science, gender lore, and celebrity narratives." *Canadian Women Studies* 18 (2/3): 59–63.

Hayes, S. 1998. *The cultural contradictions of motherhood.* Boston: Yale University Press.

Human Rights Watch Report. 1995. "The fall of Srebrenica and the failure of UN peacekeeping Bosnia and Herzegovina." Available at https://www.hrw.org/sites/defa ult/files/reports/ bosnia1095web.pdf (accessed 8 August 2018).

Jacobs, J. 2017. "The memorial at Srebrenica: Gender and the social meanings of collective memory in Bosnia-Herzegovina." *Memory Studies* 10 (4): 423–439.

Joy Green, F. 2004. "Feminist mothers: Successfully negotiating the tension between motherhood as institution and experience." In A. O'Reilly (Ed.), *From motherhood to mothering: The legacy of Adrienne Rich's Of woman born* (125–136). New York: SUNY Press.

Kašić, B., Prlenda, S., Petrović, J., and Slapšak, S. 2012. *Feminist critical interventions. Thinking heritage, decolonising, crossings.* Ljubljana, Zagreb, and Belgrade: Red Athena University Press.

Kinnvall, C. 2013. "Trauma and the politics of fear: Europe at the crossroads." In N. Demertzis (Ed.), *Emotions in politics. Palgrave studies in political psychology series* (143–166). London: Palgrave Macmillan.

Kleck, M. 2006. "Working with traumatized women." In M. Fischer (Ed.), *Peacebuilding and civil society in Bosnia-Herzegovina. Ten years after Dayton* (343–355). Münster: Lit-Verlag.

Klein, M. and Riviere, J. 1962. *Love, hate, and reparation*. London: The Hoghart Press.

Korac, M. 1998. "Ethnic nationalism, wars and the patterns of social, political and sexual violence against women: The case of post-Yugoslav countries." *Identities Global Studies in Culture and Power* 5 (2): 153–181.

Kumar, K. 2012. "Mass crimes and resilience of women: A cross-national perspective." In A. Schnabel and A. Tabyshalieva (Eds.), *Defying victimhood: Women and post-conflict peacebuilding* (79–95). New York: United Nations University Press.

Leydesdorff, S. 2007. "Stories from no land: The women of Srebrenica speak out." *Human Rights Review* 8 (3): 187–198.

Licht, S. and Drakulic, S. 1996. "When the word for peace was woman: War and gender in the Former Yugoslavia." In B. Wejnert and M. Spencer (Eds.), *Women in post-communism* (111–139). Greenwich, CT/London: IAI Press.

Lineman Nelson, H. 2001. *Damaged identities: Narrative repair*. Ithaca, NY: Cornell University Press.

Miklikowska, M. 2015. "Like parent, like child? Development of prejudice and tolerance towards immigrants." *British Journal of Psychology* 107 (1): 95–116.

Močnik, N. 2017. *Sexuality after war rape: From narrative to embodied research*. New York: Routledge.

Mulalic, M. 2011. "Women's NGOs and civil society building in Bosnia-Herzegovina." *Epiphany* 4 (1): 40–55.

Nikolić-Ristanović, V. 2000. *Women, violence, and war: Wartime victimization of refugees in the Balkans*. Budapest: Central European University Press.

O'Bryan, M., Fishbein H. D., and Neal, R. P. 2004. "Intergenerational transmission of prejudice, sex role stereotyping, and intolerance." *Adolescence* 39 (155): 407–426.

O'Reilly, A. (Ed.). 2004. *Motherhood to mothering: The legacy of Adrienne Rich's of woman born*. Albany: State University of New York Press.

O'Reilly, A. 2009. *Maternal thinking: Philosophy, politics, practice*. Toronto: Demeter Press.

Paechter, C. 2007. *Being boys, being girls: Learning masculinities and femininities*. Maidenhead, UK: Open University.

Pankov M., Mihelj, S., and Bajt, V. 2011. "Nationalism, gender and the multivocality of war discourse in television news." *Media, Culture and Society* 33 (7): 1043–1059.

Papić, Ž. 1979. "Društveni položaj žene - specifičnosti i teškoće utemeljenja problema." *Žena* 3: 106–116.

Papić, Ž. 1994. "Nationalism, patriarchy and war in ex-Yugoslavia." *Women's History Review* 3 (1): 115–117.

PBS. 2018. *UN sex abuse scandal*. Available at https://www.pbs.org/wgbh/frontline/film/un-sex-abuse-scandal/ (accessed 8 August 2018).

Popov-Momčinović, Z. 2013. *Ženski pokret u Bosni I Herzegovini: Artikulacija jedne kontrakulture*. Sarajevo: Sarajevski otvoreni centar, Centar za empirijska istraživanja religije u Bosni I Herzegovini, Fondacija CURE.

Pusić, V. 1976. "O nekim aspektima uloge feminizma u suvremenom društvu." *Žena* 3: 120–124.

Ramanathapillai, R. 2006. "The politicizing of trauma: A case study of Sri Lanka." *Peace and Conflict: Journal of Peace Psychology* 12 (1): 1–18.

Ruddick, S. 1989. *Maternal thinking: Toward a politics of peace.* Boston, MA: Beacon Press.

Russell-Brown, S. 2003. "Rape as an act of genocide." *Berkeley Journal of International Law* 21 (2): 350–374.

Schirch, L. 2012. "Frameworks for understanding women as victims and peacebuilders." In A. Schnabel and A. Tabyshalieva (Eds.), *Defying victimhood: Women and post-conflict peacebuilding* (48–76). New York: United Nations University Press.

Schnabel, A. and Tabyshalieva, A. (Eds.). 2012. *Defying victimhood: Women and post-conflict peacebuilding.* Washington, DC: Brookings Institution Press.

Schnabel, A. and Tabyshalieva, A. 2012. "Forgone opportunities: The marginalization of women's contributions to post conflict peacebuilding." In A. Schnabel and A. Tabyshalieva (Eds.), *Defying victimhood: Women and post-conflict peacebuilding* (3–47). New York: United Nations University Press.

Sideris, T. 2001. "Rape in war and peace: Social context, gender, power and identity." In S. Meinjtes, A. Pillay, and M. Turshen (Eds.), *Women in post-conflict transformation* (142–157). London: Zed Books.

Simić, O. 2009. "What remains of Srebrenica? Motherhood, transitional justice and yearning for the truth." *Journal of International Women's Studies* 10 (4): 220–236.

Simić, O. 2012. "Challenging Bosnian women's identity as rape victims, as unending victims: The 'other' sex in times of war." *Journal of International Women's Studies* 13 (4): 129–142.

Skjelsbaek, I. 2006. "Victim and survivor: Narrated social identities of women who experienced rape during the war in Bosnia-Herzegovina." *Feminism and Psychology* 16 (4): 373–403.

Škrgic-Mikulić, E. 2016. *Bosnian war rape victims rue lost motherhood.* Available at http://www.balkaninsight.com/en/article/bosnian-war-rape-victims-rue-lost-motherhood-10-20-2016 (accessed 1 August 2018).

Udruženje 'Pokret Majke enclave Srebrenica I Žepa. 2017. Available at http://www.enklave-srebrenica-zepa.org/

Walsh, M. 1997. *Postconflict Bosnia-Herzegovina: Integrating women's special situation and gender perspectives in skills training and employment promotion programs.* Geneva: ILO.

Warren, K. 1990. "The power and promise of ecological feminism." *Environmental Ethics* 12 (3): 125–146.

Watson-Franke, M. 2004. "We have a mama but no papa: Motherhood in women-centred societies." In A. O'Reilly (Ed.), *Motherhood to motherhing: The legacy of Adrienne Rich's of woman born* (75–87). Albany: State University of New York Press.

Weiss, K. G. 2010. "Too ashamed to report: Deconstructing the shame of sexual victimization." *Feminist Criminology* 5 (3): 286–310.

Wenger, E. 1998. *Communities of practice: Learning, meaning and identity.* Cambridge: Cambridge University.

Yuval-Davis, N. 1997. *Gender and nation.* New York: Sage Publications.

Žarkov, D. 1995. "Gender, orientalism and the history of ethnic hatred in the Former Yugoslavia." In H. Lutz, A. Phoenix, and N. Davis Yuval (Eds.), *Crossfires: Nationalism, racism, and gender in Europe* (105–120). London: Pluto Press.

Žarkov, D. 2007. *The body of war: Media, ethnicity, and gender in the break-up of Yugoslavia.* Durham, NC: Duke University Press.

Zembylas, M. 2007a. "The politics of trauma: Empathy, reconciliation and peace education." *Journal of Peace Education* 4 (2): 207–224.

Zembylas, M. 2007b. "The affective politics of hatred: Implications for education." *Intercultural Education* 18 (3): 177–192.

Zraly, M., Rubin, S. E., and Mukamana, D. 2013. "Motherhood and resilience among Rwandan genocide-rape survivors." *Ethos: Journal of the Society for Psychological Anthropology* 41 (4): 411–439.

5 Intergenerational effects of trauma transmission and continuation of violent sexual culture

Between forgiveness and rage, forgetting and transmitting

There is a scene in Lars Feldballe-Petersen's 2017 documentary film *The Unforgiven* where Esad Landžo, convicted of war crimes and crimes against humanity at the International Criminal Tribunal for the former Yugoslavia in 1998, stands at the location of the former Čelebići prison camp, the very place where he was a guard during the war. In front of him are the men who survived his torture. It is a striking scene, representing the culmination of Landžo's journey to search for survivors and ask for their forgiveness – as it is preceded by very graphic survivor testimonies, it is almost surreal to witness this moment in such a raw, documentary format. In a carefully crafted narrative, the director follows the story of Landžo for 12 years, shifting the conversation from forgiveness on the part of the survivors to those responsible for the crimes and suffering. It is a rare moment to hear a perpetrator thinking and reflecting extensively on forgiveness, as Landžo does in the film.

In an interview with Alison Rice (2002, 283), Julia Kristeva – one of the most important thinkers on the topic of forgiveness – shares a similar, though unrelated example of a young adult who joined the Nazi party during World War II and participated in torturing prisoners in camps. After a few decades, after serving a prison sentence and attempting to (re)start a normal life, he begins to be haunted by his past; no longer a component of the agonistic and chaotic war machinery, he is overwhelmed by conscious thoughts and self-reflection concerning the crimes he committed. In her writing on forgiveness, Kristeva insists that criminals can be and must be forgiven, but only after reparations have been made and crimes punished. Using the example mentioned above, she explains:

> I tell him that his acts will be judged and punished, that he will be asked for explanations, that he will be asked to make reparations in various ways. But I also tell him that he will be permitted – and this is where forgiveness will intervene – to transform himself, to free himself from this stigma. He will not be allowed to forget, but to start over.
>
> (Kristeva in Rice 2002, 283)

In this way, both Kristeva and Feldballe-Petersen acknowledge the occurrence of trauma among perpetrators, and with this the necessity to humanize and consequently reintegrate these perpetrators into society. Both cases describe what Derrida calls "conditional forgiveness": while the perpetrator asks for forgiveness out of regret for his deeds, he simultaneously seeks to be free of his own trauma as a survivor. For Derrida, however, "real" forgiveness is granted by the survivor (victim), even and especially when the accused does not ask for it, does not show regret, or even insists on denying responsibility and proclaiming his innocence despite the evidence. Therefore, the guilt of the perpetrator is acknowledged; though he remains guilty and does not transform, he is nonetheless forgiven (Derrida 2000).

In this way, Derrida places the power in the perpetrator's hands: forgiveness is subject to the perpetrator's willingness to feel remorse and apologize, and this conditions how survivors will forgive. And while in *The Unforgiven* we know from the start that Landžo's statement is pre-determined – he wants to apologize – the response from the survivors is more ambiguous. The idea of meeting the person who subjected you to torture, with the intention of forgiving that person in an attempt at mutual exchange and postwar rehumanization, seemed incomprehensible to some who were invited to meet with Landžo. On the other hand, a curiosity or belief among some survivors held that doing so would change the power relationship and help them to move on in the healing process. While some of the invited survivors were willing to forgive but lacked the strength to meet Landžo in person, others were motivated by the desire to tell him to his face of the pain he caused – a pain that they still live with.

When they actually meet, however, the anticipated goals of the meeting change. While contemplating the meeting from the safe space of their homes allowed the survivors to imagine and project the process of apology and forgiveness – with Landžo as the perpetrator and the survivors granting him forgiveness – the actual meeting turned out to be much more challenging. Regardless of their reasons – whether their motivation was moral or to improve their own mental well-being – the survivors *made a decision to forgive*; the physical encounter, however, challenged them in the *act of forgiving*. Although Landžo describes how his own violent past haunts him in ways that are similar to the experiences of the survivors of his aggression, and while he expresses remorse several times throughout the film, viewers can detect hesitancy in the survivors' reaction to this unconventional apology. Their mistrust is expressed in their body language and in their reflections of someone who, despite his apparent remorse, is not to be fully trusted.

For Landžo, serving a prison sentence and eventually receiving forgiveness from survivors would presumably bring him some relief; forgiveness might lessen future PTSD symptoms on an individual level and, on a collective level, represent a step toward reconciliation and justice. However, the end of the film leaves the viewer questioning if this is true – if apology and forgiveness have really brought any relief or have any power in reconciliation and (social) recovery in the aftermath of the war.

Forgiving the forgivable is very easy, says Derrida, but what if *some offenses are just unforgivable*? (Card 2002). Arendt wrote of the necessity of punishment in her forgiveness paradigms: "men are unable to forgive what they cannot punish," while at the same time they are "unable to punish what has turned out to be unforgivable" (Arendt 1958, 241). Arendt is generally concerned about the question of execution as *true punishment* for crimes that are eventually deemed unforgivable; for her, the negotiation of justice through the legal system and punishment are necessary prerequisites for forgiveness. With the establishment of international criminal courts and truth and reconciliation commissions to provide systematic legal procedures for defining, recognizing, and punishing serious human rights violations and crimes against humanity, these requirements seem to have generated a response. For Derrida, however, forgiveness should not be confused, determined by, or equated with political and/or legal processes.

Along with Derrida, Vladimir Jankélévitch (in Looney, 2015), Paul Ricoeur (1973), and Aurel Kolnai (1973) understand forgiveness in primarily moral and ethical terms. In the words of Kolnai, it is "unjustified or pointless" (1973, 99) if a "change of heart" (1973, 97) does not occur within the one who has been forgiven. Jankélévitch insists that forgiveness must involve a "real relation with another person" (in Looney 2015, xxi). Ideally, forgiveness would be a mutual (survivor-perpetrator), multidimensional (survivors-perpetrators; individuals-collectives; personal-institutional), and intersectional process that has as its goal the assertion of responsibility and payment of reparations. In this kind of relationship, while the person must be forgiven, the crime is not. According to Julia Kristeva, while the actions of criminals are trialed and punished in the social space, forgiveness should remain an intimate and private human interaction. In contexts so complicated and painful for survivors – where the processes of transitional and restorative justice are so fragile and subject to failure – this intimate encounter is a rather challenging task.

In Western preoccupation with "closure" (for more, see in van der Veer 1998) and as an individual approach to healing for survivors, it has been argued that forgiveness is important in moving on and growing emotionally in the aftermath of conflict. It is often encouraged in psychotherapeutic processes as it presumably allows the one who mourns to transform and release negative emotions, especially guilt, anger, remorse, dread, and anxiety (Cerney 1988), replacing them with more constructive and positive feelings of compassion, even love, toward the perpetrators (Cosgrove & Konstam 2008). Clinical psychologists agree that this is a deliberate and volitional process that only happens over time. It is a process that demands acceptance and change – in the emotional, cognitive, and behavioral perceptions of justice and one's world (see Webb et al. 2017). Those who stress the importance of forgiveness reportedly have fewer and less intense traumatic symptoms and experience an overall improvement in well-being (Brown 2003; Thompson 2005). By this account, forgiveness is a step toward recovery for those who have been wronged.

For Margaret Holmgren (1993), who has argued for unilateral forgiveness, the process of forgiving is all about the victims – they were insulted and humiliated;

therefore, only victims themselves can restore their self-respect and regain the desired social status destroyed by transgressors. As a successful outcome of such "genuine forgiveness" (Holmgren 1993, 345), the victim opens "himself up to positive emotional states such as love, joy, excitement and gratitude." Upon truly forgiving the offender, the victim-survivor also benefits from an internal peace attained by the fact that the incident is over and no longer preoccupies her mind. Not only is this peace of mind desirable in itself, it also allows the victim to concentrate on her own positive pursuits (Holmgren, ibid.).

In her distinction between the private and public spheres of forgiveness, Kristeva emphasizes that the most important part of the process is the work of first *forgiving oneself*, which allows for personal rebirth and the "optimistic advancement toward new horizons" (in Rice 2002, 280). Hannah Arendt also ascribes a great deal to the religious responsibility of forgiving others or *forgiving oneself* before God, which, although not necessarily the best choice empirically, may be the option that allows survivors to move on with their lives. As sociopolitical and legal procedures fail to provide just and transparent reparations to survivors, and the prolonged responses seem to rely on amnesia and the excuses of outdated cases in the courts, forgiving oneself is for many survivors the only option. One survivor tells me:

> I no longer expect that anyone will apologize. I am no longer seeking this. But I have spent years blaming myself – not for the rape, but for me being unable to heal, to recover, to move on with my life. But now I forgive myself my struggle.
>
> (L, Central Bosnia 2019)

However, Robin May Schott (2004, 208–209) mentions that the empirical accounts of war-rape survivors do not ascribe to forgiveness a fundamental role in the recovery process after all. Listing some of the most complex examples, she asks if the pressure to forgive is in the end not merely a burden, as none of the arguments for it are very compelling. She briefly discusses the idea of replacing forgiveness with other terms, such as witnessing (in Card 2002) or righteous indignation (Herman 1992). The survivor abandons the fantasy of revenge as a means of regaining a sense of power but continues to hold the perpetrators accountable for their crimes in her quest for justice (Herman 1992, 189). In any case, it is important that every individual survivor decide what she wants to forgive and what long-term (most probably positive) outcomes she anticipates in doing so.

In the writings of Ricoeur and Derrida, forgiveness in the context of reconciliation ideologies can be applied on two levels. On the individual level, survivors and preparators strive to discard their war-roles in order to build new relationships and a new social order. The process of forgiveness from individual to individual is very emotional, personal, and intimate, but also unpredictable and potentially deeply retraumatizing. On the second level, the processes of forgiveness are more instrumentalized: they constitute a matter in current political efforts to respond to the economic, administrative, and legal aspects of the past's traumatic heritage. Forgiving a perpetrator as a fellow human being is therefore only one level of the process, and perhaps because it is more concrete, it is easier for the survivors; it shows, as in the Landžo case, the establishment of an empathetic understanding on which to build.

On the other hand, it is much more challenging – yet not so often discussed – to forgive *the system* that allowed such crimes to happen, and which allows these crimes to remain unpunished. One of the survivor's explains:

> For the war, I somehow came to terms, that it was chaos. It is hard to comprehend, but it was a war. And now, we live in peace – everyone who denies what happened are criminals, aren't they? Everyone who helps to cover criminals is a criminal? This is what I cannot forgive.
>
> (J56, Sarajevo 2018)

As narrated silences, instrumentalized forgiveness is strategically planned and navigated by interested social agents and political bodies. As such, it loses its purity, according to Derrida. Forgiveness should remain exceptional, extraordinary (Derrida 2000, 107–108): "forgiveness projects" developed through systematic and intentional collective projects (whether at the community, national, or international level) are therefore trivialized and do not represent real forgiveness. However, for forgiveness to remain an intimate and private act of human interaction, there must be a clear division between criminals and their crimes. While the criminals are to be forgiven, the crimes must not be forgotten, especially in an unstable, corrupt, and manipulated postconflict context such as Bosnia-Herzegovina. Failing to understand the political dynamics, after war social development, and collective wrongdoing of such mass crimes, as well as their historical and contextual uniqueness, would be dangerous. Granting forgiveness to wrongdoers in such a context risks conveying the wrong messages – that the perpetrators can return to normal social life and sometimes even regain political power.

If the criminals' former crimes are not punished – that is, if the crimes are not acknowledged as such by law – then where is the guarantee that, given a similar sociopolitical environment, any future crimes will be punished? In a sociopolitical situation where convicted war criminals return to their own countries as war heroes, forgiveness might allow them to reestablish their political agendas. What prevents these former criminals from continuing their ideological agenda, which could very well be the old plan, reorganized and placed within the new postwar social order? As the context of a postconflict or transitional society differs significantly from the prewar context, collectives might not at first recognize the patterns that signal a continuation of the dangerous and radical ideologies that, should they be allowed to develop, might lead to the same devastating policies. In fact, just such a scenario has unfolded with several convicted war criminals who have returned to their homelands after serving their sentences.

While the theoretical proposition of separating criminals from their crimes might have some moral weight as a means of enabling a sustainable peace and the community's willingness to reconcile, there is a dearth of theoretical and empirical knowledge concerning postwar recovery and the social reintegration of perpetrators. While we remain preoccupied with the silence of survivors, we overlook the silence of perpetrators. For now, as we tend to elaborate forgiveness, we do this without strong evidence as to who is to be forgiven, and if that person even wants to be forgiven. This knowledge would be essential to our understanding of forgiveness – not only as a one-sided decision with the goal of self-recovery but also as a relationship with others. When thinking of how to forgive, either conditionally or unconditionally, we mostly speculate about the perpetrators' attitude, imagining how they would ask for and accept forgiveness and how they would live with being (or not) forgiven.

The rare case of Esad Landžo shows that the process of forgiveness is way more complicated, even when asking for forgiveness and eventually being forgiven; moreover, it questions the very idea of forgiveness and its power in one's individual and general social recovery from trauma. Despite a lack of evidence, at least in the case of the Bosnian war, writings on forgiveness often assume the preexistence of a relationship between those who forgive and those who ask for forgiveness. The only relationship that most of the survivors who participated in my research have with the perpetrators is when they met them, behind glass, in the very formal and impersonal setup of court. Some of the survivors who experienced rapes by several individuals have only an imagined image of the perpetrator. One of the survivors told me that, given the chance, she would avoid meeting the man who raped her:

> I do not want to see him as an ordinary man. For instance, how he cuts the grass in the garden. For me, he will always be only a rapist, I cannot see him as a family man, I do not want to know anything about him.
>
> (A, Sarajevo 2019)

I asked her how her ideas about him might change if she could see him in everyday situations, such as queuing in the bank, or holding his grandson's hand while walking him to kindergarten. She responds:

> Of course, it is very probable that he is something like this! Look, I am, I am not just a rape survivor, I am a grandmother – why do you think he would not have a normal life? For him it is even easier I think! But I do not want to know or see him like this. For me, he is not a normal man, only a man sick in his head can do this to a woman. I don't know what I would feel if I were to see him on the street.
>
> (A, Sarajevo 2019)

As the testimonies of survivors are now publicly available through various platforms, one can learn about their struggles involving social reintegration, their attempts to return to "normal" in the aftermath of the war, and their problems associated with ostracism and social stigma. On the other hand, the lack of evidence for PTSD among perpetrators, as well as their almost complete silence, gives the impression that postwar social reintegration for the perpetrators has been easier than it was for the survivors. The absence of public remorse from the perpetrators lends credence to this assumption. While survivors want to be socially perceived as "normal" – as mothers, workers, women, and citizens – they refuse to extend these identities to the perpetrators, seeing them instead solely in their criminal "war" identity.

One survivor carries a very clear image of the man who raped her: she describes a face destroyed by years of smoking; his skin pale grey; his big "Chetnik" moustache; big belly, bad breath, and even the smell of his skin. She is aware that he looks different today, as does she, yet she cannot imagine him differently. Another survivor describes how, following the trial of the man who raped her, she cannot reconcile her memory of the man with the man she confronted in court:

> He is very old and when I first saw him, of course all the images came back. But at the same time, this man in jeans and a jacket haunted me. I walked the streets for months, wondering about the past of every man who passed me. They look so normal! But I know they must carry, some of them, bad things.
>
> (M, 2015, Central Bosnia)

Several women who tried to recall the physical appearance of the men described them as ugly, smelly, sometimes fat. One of the women described to me a very detailed image of a young man who had been about 20 years younger than her: "I felt sorry for his mother, this boy was attractive and well built. He was around the age of my son" (R, Central Bosnia, July 2018). She said that her memory of him was so strong that she would immediately recognize him today. When I responded by noting that this man would be in his fifties today – an adult man who perhaps has adolescent children – she continued:

> To me, he is innocent. I cannot think of him without thinking of my son, the older one that vanished. I was angry, and I am angry still today, but I think he was manipulated. Maybe I am trying to be angry, but I always think of my son when I think of him, I don't know why. I will never forget, but I think I forgave.
>
> (R, Central Bosnia, July 2018)

If there is no relationship between the perpetrators and survivors, as is the case of the survivors in my research, the process of forgiveness is subject to a memory of events and an image of the perpetrator that are mostly fixed in the past. In the above example, the young boy mentioned by the woman is today a man; perhaps he has a mustache and a belly; perhaps, as she remembers him, he was *only* manipulated and, like Landžo, regrets his actions and would seek forgiveness. He could be, as Arendt writes of Eichmann, just *a clown*, unable to truly understand the scope of his actions. For some survivors, dealing with the remembered image of the perpetrator, rather than the person they are today, makes the process of forgiveness easier. Without actually encountering the perpetrator, the survivors can create their own version of his identity. She can construct her own arguments for his actions, and therefore believe that he is apologetic and remorseful.

Without knowing him today, she can believe that he is, like her, haunted by the past; that he struggles in isolation and must cope with his own perpetrators' trauma. She can relate her own PTSD to that of the perpetrators. What most survivors describe is not a revenge fantasy but a fantasy of shared pain. In one of the workshops, where we reenacted an encounter with the perpetrator,[1] this *shared pain* was expressed through the survivor's imagined relationship and mother-to-mother connection with the mother of the man in question. Survivors described perpetrators as lost children; perhaps their mothers did not love them. They expressed pity before conveying rage or anger; but it was a pity reserved mostly for their mothers, not the perpetrators themselves.

The emotional response that accompanied group work discussions of rapists *as individuals* differed from discussions of the rapes as *systematic and strategically planned crimes*. In a dysfunctional postwar state, survivors could exercise forgiveness on an individual, person-to-person level, mostly in the form of an imaginary image/representation and dialogue with the perpetrator. Many war rapes survivors did not have the opportunity to meet the perpetrators, even in the official setting of the trial, and so their current attitude toward forgiveness or the possibility of dialogue is speculation. The belief that the perpetrator does in fact feel regret and remorse gives survivors hope and a belief in justice ("he must be suffering too now"). On the other hand, testifying at the trials – especially with insensitive cross-examinations – was an extremely traumatizing experience for some survivors, and in most cases the perpetrator expressed no remorse. In such cases, the survivors described feeling disappointment rather than anger or rage.

Survivors therefore often separate the *crime by the individual* from the *crime of the system*; it is much easier to connect with the individual perpetrator as a fellow human being than it is the entire ideological machine that compelled those individuals to act against each other. Not all crimes carry the same symbolic meaning and political implications; nor do the criminals operate with equal power resources. Therefore, not wanting to see the perpetrator today in everyday life helps survivors to keep the memory of the perpetrator as evil, as a wrongdoer. The rehumanization of individuals who have committed crimes could lead to accepting the system that produced them. This is the system of good and bad, of perpetrators and victims, of unequal relationships and power balances that cannot be fully understood and reapplied in the aftermath of the war. Survivors are aware that perpetrators have changed, and that some of them regret their actions, but they cannot accept this rehumanization until they have been assured that their crimes will not be forgotten or denied.

Given the long time-span of the war/postwar period, the great variety of contexts from which individual social players entered and exited the conflict, and the losses suffered by everyone, simplifying the perpetrators' motives and "recovery" in the aftermath of the conflict would be as unfair as considering the victims as collectives. What one must see in Kristeva's criminal-crime separation – and this is similar to other forms of discrimination and exclusive practices – are the structural components of dealing with justice, crime, and criminals in the aftermath of war, not the remorse and regret that comes from individuals. Retributive justice is crucial for individuals to think about forgiveness:

> It was important to witness the trial, to know that he got what he deserved. But I do not feel that I have to seek some revenge now. For me it is enough to know that he went to jail. He will now have to think about this every day and night. And I admit, I enjoy thinking of this, just a little bit. And this makes it easier for me to think to forgive him.
>
> (R67, Central Bosnia 2017)

For those survivors who know the identity of their rapists, or know where they and their families live today, legal prosecution is not just a demand for justice and reparation but also a matter of safety. The ability to move on therefore depends not only on some type of moral work, but in day-to-day relief, living a life without fear or threats – this is what a *prosecuted individual* means for the survivors. Beyond this, more emphasis is given to the structural components and symbolic meanings of criminals *and their* crimes – thought of as plural, as collective. Despite the efforts of the many scholars who have emphasized the critique of collective guilt (the nation as perpetrator, for instance), survivors do recognize that collective guilt is more important than the singular acts of individuals. From this perspective, we can see how Esad Landžo, as an individual asking for forgiveness, can in a way be easily forgiven.

What does it mean, in the end, if only one individual out of thousands apologizes, while the survivor returns to an everyday life full of divisive politics, manipulations of the war discourse, the pain and grief of having lost loved ones, and retraumatizing events such as stigmatization and ostracism? Will the perpetrator's own, individual remorse promote collective changes and spark something like collective remorse? For the apology to have an effect on the survivors' lives, the perpetrator should actively engage with the current political demands of survivors, standing by their side and fighting for their rights. In this way, perhaps, the apology would foster an empowering momentum for both sides, and thus break down the established divisions.

Arendt has problematized collective guilt in the sense that it in fact prevents prosecution, because "if everyone is guilty, nobody is, and therefore nobody can be judged" (Arendt 2003, 29). In a sense, this is how the divided ethnic entities have formed a protective mechanism to address crimes committed by its members – who are now residents of these entities – to perform as collectives, both in exaggerating victimhood and in denying or covering up the crimes. Are collectives to be held accountable for the crimes committed by their members? Should these collectives bear the collective guilt? This is very slippery terrain on which to draw conclusions and is also a destructive way for the involved parties to allow social recovery and development in the aftermath of war. However, in the end, everybody is guilty because nobody is judged, to paraphrase Arendt. "It is one of my biggest frustrations," says one of the survivors after the workshops we had with youth (2018):

> I know /name omitted/, where he lives, I can take you there now. But what can I do, widowed old *baba*? I gave my testimony and I gave his name. I got threats, but he is still not in jail.
>
> *NM: Was he ever in the process?*
>
> Yes, already in 2004, but they wanted more papers from me. I went there seven times. What I do now, I am not afraid of threats, when they call me, and I tell his name to everyone. I told his name today to all the youths who were there, you heard me. Maybe they will succeed in bringing him to jail.

This survivor was not angry with the individual, the criminal, as such, but with the *collective* system that has its own agendas and motives for slowing down the process and protecting the individuals – embedded motives that are always used to make sense of the war in its aftermath, and which also constitute widely accepted ideological narratives.

But such *crime-related forgiveness* is not only about perpetrators as a collective, nor is it related only to crimes committed during the war. This level of forgiveness is only possible with the constructive collaboration of the state, the legislative system, and the involvement of all parties. Given the current political circumstances of the country, unstable, corrupted, and divisive, this is a rather unrealistic demand. The questions that both Card and Arendt address are therefore not in the nature of the crimes or in the ability of the survivors to forget. In the case of survivors of sexual violence in Bosnia-Herzegovina, it is the state institutions and governing political bodies that make the crimes unforgivable. This furthermore gives those individuals with power the opportunity to avoid being held responsible for not acting on and responding to the survivors' demands. When the memory culture of "unforgivability" is established, any unprosecuted crimes are fixed in history.

While it is true that different levels and systems of intercultural coexistence in the aftermath of war might occur with the help of individual and person-related forgiveness, long-term and stable reconciliation is only possible when state authorities work toward *collective and crime-related forgiveness*. In this sense, we should perhaps turn around Arendt's idea and consider making *everyone in the collective guilty*. When everyone in the collective is guilty, we acknowledge individuals as social actors in the postconflict environment as being guilty on a broad spectrum, not simply the perpetrator-victim binary: bystanders, as those politically supporting those responsible; witnesses who are satisfied with others speaking on their behalf; and finally, the offspring (of everyone in the aftermath despite their role in the war) as potential perpetrators. These are all potentially secondary victims and/or perpetrators – sometimes they are both.

The range of emotions that survivors feel toward the perpetrator as an individual (pity, ability to empathize) and as a collective (anger, frustration) is interesting because the promotion and encouragement of forgiveness by different stakeholders, peacebuilders, and international interveners in the aftermath of the violence often assumes that survivors face a choice between revenge or forgiveness. One's only choice, therefore, is to either dwell on the past and risk getting enmeshed in the cycles of hate that eventually lead to self-destruction, or to leave the past behind and move forward toward a better future. The pressure of forgiveness presses victims to

> take an undemanding, or even a forgiving stance, even where this frustrates their needs for vindication or forecloses any of the varieties of vindication that might satisfy their needs to have their dignity restored, their suffering acknowledged, or their losses compensated.
>
> (Brudholm & Grøn 2011, 19)

Holmgren emphasizes that forgiveness does not exclude feelings of anger and grief. Cutting off the experience of such destructive emotions denies an integral part of the victim's humanity; it "deprives herself of an opportunity to understand the incident and treats herself in a psychologically destructive manner" (Holmgren 1993, 343). Forgiveness is so strongly attached to the moral image of victimhood that the motivations of those survivors refusing to forgive are seldom considered seriously. When accepted as another legitimate and acknowledged response from the victims, the resentment involved in forgiveness is not necessarily due to a desire for revenge, but is also the result of a stubborn persistence that these crimes be acknowledged. When looking at the field of war rape policies today, and their levels of international juridical and sociopolitical recognition, we should not forget that these changes are the result of survivors who were not willing to simply forgive, forget, and move on.

Eliminating emotions that are considered "destructive" – such as hate, vengeance, and rage – is done mostly in the interest of peacebuilding efforts and to avoid sparking retributive violence. However, while forgiveness may be beneficial for society as a whole, expressing rage and anger is a healthy way for survivors to vent their trauma (Brudholm & Rosoux 2009, 105). Yet, the safe places where therapeutic support is offered to survivors have not considered working on these emotions as a means to better their psychological well-being. While several authors and clinicians have argued that anger and revenge fantasies are part of the healing and relief processes, these feelings also have the dangerous potential to set in motion a downward spiral of violence that "traps people in cycles of revenge, recrimination, and escalation" (Minow 1998, 10).

At a workshop in Sarajevo in 2015 in which we constructed short scenes and situations for survivors to explore their relationship toward both forgiveness and rage or revenge, most survivors rejected the staging of any situation involving revenge, even though it would only be a part of the revenge fantasy. That they neglected to think of any type of revenge suggests that, in this group, forgiveness was not perceived as a noble and morally appreciated human value; rather because they felt that the crimes were so unforgivable, the greatest strength could be shown not in forgiving to move on but in moving on without entertaining a revenge fantasy. At another workshop (Central Bosnia 2015), I shared with the survivors a fantasy penalty by Claudia Card (1996) that involves the surgical removal of the rapist's penis. They responded by exchanging a couple of local jokes that allowed them to join the fantasy, albeit briefly. But along with Card, they agreed that what is more important is the sociopolitical and symbolic significance of rape, its use in conflict, and the current manipulation and abuse of survivors' memories, testimonies, and needs.

Rather than a desire to emasculate the rapist, or the belief that this act could – if only as a performance staged in a safe space – bring them relief, if not justice, they felt disgust and general pity for the perpetrator in a very heterosexual, biologized, and gendered (masculine: fearless, courageous) way. Staging these encounters showed once again that the rapist, the very concrete perpetrator, is in fact the least important actor for them when it comes to questions of forgiveness and rage. Perhaps this is similar to the puzzled reaction of the survivors in Landžo's case, in which they could partly forgive him as a person, as an individual. Survivors in the film and the survivors in my workshops could differentiate between the perpetrator as the executor of the crimes and war as the institution that inflicts those crimes. One survivor explains why she does not feel the need to seek vengeance against or forgive the perpetrator as an individual:

> It's very hard. I can recall his face and I will never be able to forget this. But to me, thinking to cut off his penis is pointless. What does it change? I have a trust that my good God will punish him, if ours will not. And those are the ones I feel angry about. Those who ordered. What makes me angry is that maybe he will be punished one day, but that will never be.
>
> (R60, Northern Bosnia 2018)

Therefore, while personal transformation might lead to forgiving the act of rape, righteous indignation is also a very common response among survivors, particularly in relation to current injustices and the general political stance toward rape survivors. In *Trauma and Recovery* (1992), Judith Herman notes that anger is in most cases directed not only to the perpetrators, but also toward those silent supporters and bystanders who failed to intercede. This includes especially family members, friends, and a general society that has failed to address, understand, and respond to the current needs of survivors. One of the survivors explained:

> I am not angry at the man who raped me, I do not even remember his face, or anything. It is hard to be angry, and also to forgive. But I cannot forgive those who gave orders. I cannot forgive those who could, but did not, protect us. And mostly those who do not do anything to protect us today. This really makes me angry.
>
> (R60, Central Bosnia 2018)

But it seems to me that, even if survivors do experience anger and rage, expressing these emotions openly is often taboo; they fear that they too will be seen as perpetrators. There is a tendency to move in all ways away from the perpetrators: physically, symbolically, and metaphorically. Feelings of aggression and anger make them feel that they are no different than the perpetrators – and they want to be not only different, but better. Some of the survivors felt that forgiveness was a power that they could wield against the perpetrators, with satisfaction being derived from the assumed suffering of the perpetrator when being forgiven (from fieldnotes, July 2018):

> When women start to describe how they forgave, I can see how their power becomes embodied, like this would be a superpower, a strength, that this is something that might perhaps be taken away when subjected to violence but can now be used against the perpetrators – not the perpetrators in the physical sense, in the sense of their live presence, but the perpetrator as he exists in their imagination, their own image of him. Some of the women were extremely excited to imagine situations where they would encounter the perpetrators and would be asked for forgiveness. It is almost as if there is some type of sweet enjoyment in this projection. They liked this exercise, we spent a long time in this conversation, and they were very engaged.
>
> (July 2018)

For the survivors, forgiveness has been often tied to their faith and commitment to their religion or God. But this keeps her in another subordinate position, and the perpetrators continue their historical injustice victoriously. For the perpetrator, expressing remorse and asking for forgiveness might help reduce their sentences. For the survivor, on the other hand, it is always a type of sacrifice (Brudholm & Rosoux 2009, 45–46). While the remorseful actions of the perpetrators can benefit them both socially and politically, victory for the survivor involves primarily moral satisfaction and, perhaps, internal peace – only rarely is there financial compensation. When forgiveness in the form of "institutional forgetfulness" (Minow 1998, 15) sacrifices justice to enable survivors to coexist with unpunished perpetrators, we risk supporting the culture of silence and impunity, blaming the victims, and treating the victims as completely disempowered and powerless individuals. With this I do not say that forgiveness as such, in its moral and/or religious capacity, should be disputed; rather, we should strive for such values, realizing also that it is only possible and just to achieve such noble ends when combined with justice and an effective judicial system.

For rape survivors, forgiving the "unknown" perpetrator can be dangerous. War rape is, more than any other war crime, subject to denial and disavowal, and the survivor to social repercussions and stigmatization. Granting forgiveness in a context where (women) survivors have invested so many years and so much energy, risked their lives, exposed themselves to new threats of violence – all while the status of the war rape victim is still being disputed – could easily jeopardize current achievements in the field. For many years – and it is still happening – women have been suspected of collaborating in rapes, or of provoking them. Rather than bringing relief and helping society to reconcile, forgiveness granted from survivors to their rapists' risks confirming the existing codes of rape culture. Considering society's failure to address the social and political legacy of war, its failure to respond to transitional and retributive justice, and continuous instability in the regions, assuming a "loving stance" is naïve, if not controversial.

As pointed out earlier, forgiveness in such a context is a private matter; it is not always the product of the survivor's high ethical and moral values, but can instead result from her desire to move forward with her life, representing a first step in forgiving herself. Due to social repercussions such as stigmatization and discrimination, and the simultaneous lack of remorse expressed by the individual, the community, and even nations, the suppression of negative and destructive emotions is not the result of the survivor's psychological inability to work through her pain, but is instead a tactic that allows her to continue living in a toxic and discouraging sociopolitical postwar situation. The decision to forgive, but at the same time to forget "those times," allows some survivors to focus on the here and now. Surrounded by their family members, children, and grandchildren, they intentionally work to forget the past:

> The pain is here every day. This is why when my grandkids are around it is so hard for me. When they visit me, I think like them: I see them growing and look forward to their future. When they are not around, I remember again. I would only like to think about today, not anymore about the past.
>
> (S, Northeast Bosnia, March 2019)

I could see the connection between an inability to forgive that is the result of collective failure (as a state) and the striving to forgive among those who see forgiveness as part of their own mental and psychological recovery. In several conversations, I encountered the rage of survivors who had begun to believe that the idea of "forgiveness" had been imposed upon them. Though it originates in a very noble philosophical paradigm, the empirical manifestations of forgiveness are subjected to political manipulation and politicized processes of remembrance and memory ("reparations"). Rather than responding to the needs of survivors, these processes serve the long-term plans of the current elites: either to deny and cover their own involvement in the crimes or to ensure their existing power and control.

In contexts where most individuals have received no reparations or public recognition of their losses, forgiveness must be studied from the perspective of repressed emotions. Most of the survivors simply do not have a space and/or capacity – in physical and metaphorical sense – to express rage, disappointment, frustrations, and powerlessness in their fight against the system. I can observe the correlation between the unwillingness to forgive among those who have (re) gained powerful positions – mostly in their own organizations, but also as participants in international events, campaigns, and projects – and the higher forgiveness of those who are more dependent and less informed, and consequently less vocal and publicly resistant. Among the latter, forgiveness is strongly correlated with the desire to forget. In this sense, forgiveness is not so much an empowering strength or special moral capability of survivors, but rather an indication of surrender. Forgiveness is connected to political change; since this is not happening, survivors want to forget and move on.

At the same time, the political memory agenda – which in a divided society is aggressive and intrusive as it competes among different groups of survivors – is performed without the collaboration or input of survivors and is not in their interest. Thus, for survivors, forgetting is almost impossible. Given the corrupt and politicized nature of the national juridical system, survivors fear that forgiveness – accompanied by remorseful perpetrators – will only lead to forgetting, denying, and perhaps even repeating the same crimes. Trials, writes Booth (2001, 779), are "forums of resistance" to free perpetrators. They are a venue for "seeking the victory of the memory of justice over the will to forget, for seeking, in a sense, the rule of law. Justice and memory resist the passage of time and deny to it any power of moral/legal absolution" (ibid.).

With "restorative forgetting," Booth places the desire to "move on" at the center of transitional justice, granting the victims a kind of "compensation" and acknowledgment. They survivors shall not be abandoned for the sake of a common future – a future that is usually promoted through amnesty, or forgetting (Booth 2001, 779). Juridical recognition of crimes and official remembrance of those crimes prevents those who vanished from being forgotten, which constitutes an essential step in building a new life in the aftermath of atrocities (Booth 2001, 787). Restoration of law and justice and its importance in the healing process are, in Booth's view, essential preconditions for forgiveness and reconciliation. But like everyone else, in the corrupted and divided postconflict society, survivors as well, might manipulate within the retribution and punishment process – sometimes just in an illusionary hope to regain their loses – and in this way perpetuate further social divisions. Booth warns that survivors should not be left behind and that we, as a civil society, owe them retribution and remembrance.

This happens only rarely, however, as many countries struggle to deal with the overwhelming legacy and impact of the mass atrocities. The process of forgiving, therefore, is often dependent on grassroots initiatives and the active engagement and enthusiasm of individuals and/or survivors. The decision to "forgive" is thus also related to a failed juridical system: survivors decide to forgive to overcome resentment and hatred toward the transgressor because they have given up waiting for the state to act. The only way they can start their own, individual psychological recovery is by separating the restorative justice process – whether run by the state or the international community – from their own efforts to "move on" and create a common future. While waiting for state institutions and the juridical system to work on restorative justice, many survivors end up disappointed and, despite their own priorities, decide to forgive as the only way to start moving forward in their own private lives. In this matter, forgiveness is thus a pragmatic rather than a moral decision.

Although scholars and practitioners distinguish very clearly between *forgiving* and *forgetting*, equating these two processes, or interchanging one for the other, is common among survivors. To be able to cope with PTSD symptoms, lack of medical assistance, financial challenges, social repercussions, and numerous other issues that women must face every day, forgetting is in fact their first desire. One survivor explained to me how she became alienated from collective memory and justice projects as she felt that her contribution (giving her testimony at court in 2005) is now owned by more powerful and social institutions and agents that can actually influence the changes in this regard. Between forgiving and forgetting, she says

> I have no interest in forgiving. If you set me in front of those who com-manded crimes against us, or this one man who inflicted all this torture and pain on me and my family, why would I forgive? What would be the benefit of this? I was waiting for so long for this country to do something for us, to bring these people to justice, but they do not care. For this, I had to find my own way how to live with this, and I found it in trying to forget.
>
> (M47, March 2019)

I recorded similar "I no longer care" attitudes with others, usually in the context of self-protection. In one group conversation (Northeast Bosnia, July 2018), sur-vivors agreed that forgiveness is needed only when it helps them to move on with their lives. They expressed disappointment in the state and in the frustratingly long processes and generally unsatisfying outcomes of national and international trials. I noticed how a couple of survivors became extremely anxious when ques-tions of forgiveness arose. I met with one of these survivors some months later, and asked her to reflect on her reaction at this workshop:

> I feel the pressure to do something because no one else is doing anything. I feel the pressure from others, but listen, R /.../, she can say that God will pun-ish them, but what if I don't believe in God anymore? I lost everyone from my family, and I will never be the same as I was, and you tell me to forgive. Why is this even a question?
>
> (M46, Northeast Bosnia 2019)

I also noticed that many survivors understood their trial testimonies as their own individual contributions to combat amnesia and forgetting. However, as there is now an abundance of institutionalized remembrance practices and activists' projects, they no longer feel it necessary to continue this struggle. In light of increased awareness of testifying against crimes against humanity and a gener-ally much more effective information system, the debate on forgiveness and for-getting processes among survivors and their impact on individual and collective recovery should be further developed. To ease the trauma and PTSD symptoms, and to decrease the likelihood of retraumatization every time a survivor is asked to repeat her testimony, we should rely more on digitalized recording systems for testimonies that need only be collected once. Like it is now believed that for-giveness will bring peace to survivors' life and help them to move on, forgetting might as well be important component in healing and successful recovering. As a result of today's efficient methods of reporting, collecting, storing, and distributing information and data on crimes against humanity (or general violations of human rights), individual forgetting and collective amnesia are not exclusive.

Forgetting for the sake of individual recovery contradicts the persistent will to tell the truth, which is strongly associated with the ability to forgive. While anger and frustration are often responses to denial, silence, and ignorance, truth-telling evokes positive and hopeful feelings that furthermore evoke feelings related to Derrida's idea of "pure forgiveness" and a genuine desire to move on in a reconciled manner. Survivors often claim that they would be able to move on with their lives free of anger and disappointment if only the "truth" were to be recognized by the leading political parties (from field notes, 2017). Survivors have participated in truth-telling processes as they believed that doing so would bring them emotional relief. At the same time, they were promised that their testimonies were important both in searching for the truth and, afterward, in peace building and reconciliation processes.

Cases in which survivors have left the court retraumatized – or even exposed to threats – are not rare. David Mendeloff (2009, 595) discusses denying victims the opportunity to achieve justice or heal their psychological and emotional wounds through a truth-telling process that perpetuates cycles of violence. Most transitional justice studies second this causal logic between truth-telling and the positive benefits of reconciliation, including breaking the cycle of violence and preventing new conflicts. However, I am not certain that this is the case when we view these transitional justice processes from the perspective of war rapes and their long-term legacy. I am pessimistic not only because of the interest in denying crimes to protect perpetrators from official political institutions and bodies, but also how the formats of the social repercussions help to deny the very existence of the space for the truth-telling in many contexts by blaming and shaming the survivors. The fact that we insist on the narrative of silenced survivors despite the solid evidence that has been gathered, is one of such crimes supporting mechanisms that we all collaborate in.

In the context of war-rape survivors, there are several empirical constraints that can overshadow the psychological and emotional benefits of truth-telling. While transitional justice scholars argue that truth-telling provides victims with a sense of justice that is essential in breaking the cycle of violence, reducing anger, and minimizing the desire for vengeance, the alternative – the denial and lack of opportunities for survivors to speak – generates frustration and a sense of injustice and risks fueling the desire for violent retribution (Mendelhoff 2009, 599). In such context, transitional justice is often seen to exist in a safe vacuum that would provide survivors a welcoming, loving, and supportive environment.

However, many survivors have indicated that being abandoned by the people they counted on in the aftermath of the war, particularly their adult children, has harmed them even more than the traumatic events. Many start the process of testifying because they believe in forgiveness as a mutual process that includes remorse from the perpetrators, shifting stigmatizing and ostracizing social responses to supportive and understanding relationships. Survivors state that they engage in testifying and processes of forgiveness and reconciliation mostly because of the future of their children and grandchildren; because their own hatred will endure among future generations, leading eventually to another war. If many of the survivors strive to forgive as a means to improve their own well-being, awareness that vengeance can harm their offspring provides an even greater incentive. Choosing forgiveness over rage gives survivors the (illusory) sense that their memories of brutality and cruelty are safely in the past and that subsequent generations will not have to experience the same.

As the general conditions of life in the aftermath of war are neither good nor optimistic, facing the awful truths of the past would not necessarily break the cycle of victimization and the desire for revenge. To participate in the social contract of not repeating their past traumas, survivors *choose a moral idea of forgiveness* that is in fact an empirical will to forget and silence the pain. I claim that, as long as the idea of forgiveness enjoys respect among most survivors, they will continue to feel that they have been fooled by being asked to forgive and receiving nothing in return. For this they have built the belief that, while their will to forgive will not be repaid by remorse from the perpetrators or public admissions of guilt, it will at least ensure that future generations will experience a reconciled and shared life. In this vein, it is perhaps more productive to talk about forgiveness not as a real, performed relationship between survivors and perpetrators, but as an ideological myth to believe in for a peaceful future. Therefore, what matters is not how forgiveness is lived in everyday life but how it is communicated through the collective memory.

Trauma transmission, collective memory, and the continuation of (sexualized) violence

At the beginning of 2019, I had the opportunity to receive a small donation from a group of Danish tourists who had visited Bosnia-Herzegovina the previous summer and been deeply touched by the remains of the war and the war stories and experiences that the local people had shared with them. Knowing how donations worked behind the scenes – one cannot track how such money is spent – I expressed my hesitancy to simply transfer the money to one of the associations that works with survivors. After a couple of conversations with one of the women, we came up with the idea of using the money to organize a trip to Foča. A group of young people would join the survivors in exploring the places where atrocities had taken place. Among these were some of the most notorious, such as Karaman's house in Miljevina and the Partizan gym in Foča. The group of survivors welcomed the idea, as did the Post-Conflict Research Centre from Sarajevo, which helped to recruit the group of youngsters. On June 26, on the occasion of the International Day in Support of the Victims of Torture, we confirmed the trip. I took over the logistics involved with the event while a group of five survivors discussed how and what to share with the youngsters.

Throughout the day, the survivors repeatedly stated that what happened in these places should never be forgotten, and because "we are dying, one by one" it is now the responsibility "of the young people to keep this memory and ensure that such horrible things will never happen again" (from the fieldnotes, 2019). In contrast to the mainstream narrative of silence that I have approached critically in previous sections, this one group of survivors was extremely vocal. Prior to our workshop, I witnessed threats from locals, and arrogant, mocking comments from the police that was in charge of securing the commemoration that survivors organized, commemorating International Day for the Elimination of Sexual Violence in Conflict, on June 19, in Foča. Despite the threats, they keep fearlessly advocating for the "cancer of Bosnian memory" (N54, referring to the town of Foča and the region of Podrinje in general) and they immediately confirmed collaboration on the workshop without any hesitation.

The event brought together two generations – the generation of survivors, which has for a long time been engaged in sharing circles and public activism in relation to the restorative justice process, and the generation of young, Sarajevo-based people who are generally interested in postconflict reconstruction, collective memory, and restorative justice. The backgrounds of both groups are very important, as such a trip would not necessarily be possible with a randomly selected secondary school cohort, for instance, nor with a randomly selected group of survivors. Yet, both groups had specific reasons for appreciating this encounter, both in terms of meeting war-rape survivors and in visiting places where a large number of women were detained specifically for the purpose of rape. This group of young people had never visited Karaman's house before, nor had they participated in any commemoration activities with the survivors of war rape. At a time when survivors are still working hard to establish memorials and to mark the locations of rape atrocities around the country, this event promised to be a thought-provoking starting point in (re)considering the role of the (traumatic) collective memory in the continuation of sexual violence. While keeping the memory alive is crucial and central to the lives of survivors, questions remain as to how such memory dialogues "educate" younger generations.

After visiting Karaman's house and the Partizan gym, we left to visit the mosque in Foča, where we held a short reflective workshop. To navigate the debate that followed our visit, I suggested using the snail model of "Breaking cycles of violence, building resilience," developed by the STAR team at Eastern Mennonite University. This model offers a general overview of individual and collective trauma, common responses, and suggestions for breaking the violent cycles related to unaddressed and unhealed traumas. All participants were divided into smaller groups, and each group consisted of both survivors and young people. The model proposes different stages toward reconciliation (for instance mourning, confronting fears, memorialization, practicing tolerance, engaging the offender, etc.), and I asked each group to identify the stage at which their community is currently situated, and to list and describe the concrete actions that are being taken in relation to this. The survivors pointed optimistically to the penultimate step prior to achieving reconciliation – "integrating trauma into new self and/or group identity" – while the youth noted that society is still at the level of mere acknowledgment, namely mourning and memorializing.

To a certain extent, this can be explained by the fact that these youth had only recently been exposed to (and perhaps also personally interested in) the collective memory and political discourse related to the legacy of the war. In the meantime, for the survivors – and particularly for this group – reconciliation and personal/collective healing work has been going on for more than two decades. In addition, the entire process toward reconciliation – specifically memorialization – is very generationally specific (see Barsalou & Baxter 2007, 4). While those who survived or witnessed the atrocities memorialize in order to mourn and to seek truth, reconciliation, and social recovery, the postwar generation is expected to witness and participate in those practices in order to learn and project the lessons of the past onto their future. For the survivors, achieving justice is one of the most important incentives for insisting on certain memorial narratives; for young people, it is important to understand not only who the victims and perpetrators were, or how many and which people were killed, but how individual human beings, anywhere in the world, including themselves, can reach the point of committing such atrocities – and what they can do to prevent it.

Young people need to understand the stages and early warning signs of the process that leads to mass executions. And this is how the groups debated the step proposed in the snail model. For the survivors this involved very practical, very concrete reflections, while the youth viewed it as more of a theoretical model. While the survivors therefore heal, and are in the process of *rehabilitation*, the youth focus on *prevention*. While both generations could theoretically engage in both processes (youth in rehabilitation of transmitted traumas and survivors in prevention with the experience of violence), only recently does this seem to have become a matter of practice. The collective memory and what this collective memory communicates is therefore extremely important. While accessing evidence on how trauma is transmitted in families show that those processes are often unconscious and un-reflected, the (re)creation of the collective memory is a practice shared by the wider public, and many of the survivors (especially mothers) actively participate in it. If communicating their own experiences in their own families is unimaginable for them, then we as educators must consider how to intervene in family dynamics and the early stages of socialization with the collective memory and how to approach it critically by teaching the *literacy of collective memory*.

One of the first steps in this is to make mothers aware – informed and trained – that they can communicate their traumatic pasts by engaging with the collective memory in their homes. In the conclusion of the book I propose the necessary steps in dealing with trauma using individual psychotherapeutic and sociotherapeutic approaches that focus on the more collective work in society. Since history is often burdensome for survivors, they should be given the opportunity to focus first and fully on their own recovery, leaving the postwar generation in charge of creating the future – perhaps even without memory. However, I do not believe that this generation can create a truly alternative future if they are continuously pressured to remember the past and to engage in the remembrance practices of older generations with different agendas. Nevertheless, what is to remember from the war rapes?

As I have written elsewhere in the book, most of our global societies remain remarkably patriarchal: girls are being raised by cautionary intergenerational tales of rape and their own responsibilities in avoiding it. Susan Brison thinks of such socialization as a "postmemory of sexual violence," and "a postmemory of rape" (Brison 2002, 87). Even if we are never assaulted in childhood, the postmemory of sexual violence haunts every woman, especially when she enters adulthood. Having a memory of the of rape experience, mother–survivors fear – and sometimes anticipate – that the same will happen to their daughters. In a letter written by a survivor who participated in the July 2018 workshop, one can read:

> Dear, you are now young, and you cannot understand what war is. When you grow up, you will be a mother, you will lose sons and your daughters will be raped, if you experience war. All people are the same, take care of brotherhood and unity as the pupil of your eye. Be good. I love you.

For both the mother and her offspring, the memory of rape in the aftermath of war becomes instruction in performing gender and sexuality. The threat of rape does not end with the signed peace accord; she sees predators all around. Moreover, as many survivors joined associations, they were informed about the general rape culture – aspects of which include the abusive notions of nonconsensual sexual relationships, the obligation to sexually satisfy her spouse, and marital rape. Perhaps unsurprisingly, I recorded many testimonies in which survivors were able to recognize abusive relationships and childhood abuse only when they started to receive the psychotherapeutic support which they had sought primarily to address the war rape. This made many women aware of the male counterparts in their closest circles, and what kind of threat they might present, particularly to their daughters.

Brison (2002, 87) says that a mother's postmemories are transmitted into prememories (of her daughter's own future rape) "through early and ongoing socialization of girls and women, and both infect the actual experiences and memories of rape survivors." As opposed to postmemories – which are inherited from parents but also learned through representations in popular culture – a prememory is paradoxical as it is impossible to "remember" the future. But as an anticipation of the future rape of their daughters, the prememory is a fear that is in a future-directed state, and "a fear that is instilled by [the] postmemory of rape" (Brison 2002, 87). Both in war and peace, the stereotype and cultural determination of victims is attached to women and is passed from one woman to another in what I define as the vertical and horizontal transmission of collective memory.

Vertical transmission occurs in sharing circles of women where the peer pressure to execute cultural codes happens through discursive engagement and witnessing. One of the most discussed identities that is created partly through such vertical transmission is the collective victimhood among survivors. Although individuals enter this process with their own distinctive experience and knowledge, the sharing circles confirm, reaffirm, and exchange representations, desired and expected social roles, values, behaviors, and future projections. Similarly, in terms of collective victimhood, also transmitted are ideas of sexuality and gender. This does not mean that there is only one narrative or one set of behaviors, values, and viewpoints; rather, while variety exists, the hierarchy is established. For one to become a part of the community and to enjoy its benefits, one must comply with those viewpoints.

In *horizontal transmission*, the selected values, narratives, and beliefs that are reaffirmed in sharing circles are passed on to the next generation. This is how the stigma that is attached to women as victims of violence remains with them forever and is passed from generation to generation. From the time a girl is born, the fearful mother tells her to be careful. The girl learns about the vulnerability that is attached to her gender, and she learns this through the protection or/and fear of her mother. When mothers experience traumatic events, like war rape, they construct their identities in the aftermath according to these experiences, but not necessarily only as victims. However, when the identity label most associated with survivors is passive victim or silenced survivor, this will in one way or another affect her practice of mothering. To what extent does the transfer of her own trauma affect the socialization of gender and sexuality? Can women who were subjected to extreme sexual violence prevent transferring this violent sexual culture through their mothering?

The survivor's work lies not only in contributing her own shattered pieces of memory to create a narrative of collective trauma. To teach her children about life beyond her war experience, she must regain the memory of *what she has lived before*: her knowledge and experience. She must also acknowledge those sexual relationships, if any, that were not nonconsensual, violent, and abusive. The memory of traumatic experience tends to seize the survivor's most basic cognitive and emotional capacities, leaving her with memories of her earlier, lost life. While her shattered trust in the world and her own safety and role in it can be pieced together in the slow and protracted recovery process, the monopolistic rule of her trauma experience risks jeopardizing trauma-free child-rearing. However, one is never only fully subjected to the symptoms of her trauma; she can control certain aspects of it, particularly how to engage it in family life.

An important part of the psychosocial recovery of survivors lies not only in treating direct physical and psychological reactions, but also in learning how to render those reactions less intrusive, and "giving them the kind of meaning that enables them to be integrated into the rest of life" (Brison 2002, 54). We can look at survivors' testimonies and collective narratives as institutionalized transmissions of war rape experiences, but these do not necessarily rely on *what happened* (as it is in the case of testifying for juridical purposes); it relies rather on how a survivor *wants to be perceived* and remembered. This is particularly important when it comes to the image of a mother in the eyes of her child. Stigma and shame are attached to the survivors of war rapes; so too are the depression and hopelessness symptoms of PTSD. But mothers would prefer that their children not see this. One of the survivors tells me:

> When I remember all the pain, the suffering, I feel lost, sometimes I cry. And sometimes it is hard to hide this in front of my kids. It is better now, but I remember, it was very soon after the war, my baby was five. I have never wanted him to see me like this. I wanted him to see me smiling and to be happy, to see my love for him and that he means everything to me.
>
> (M, Central Bosnia 2018)

Mothers, with their strength, courage, virtues, and skills, would like to be seen as role models; thus, many will do anything to block the transmission of shame, guilt, powerlessness, and hopelessness. Yet, when it comes to the transmission of collective traumas, the parent's consciousness has only limited power, and every child gives up some portion of their life – whether large or small – to heal their parent's pain (Kaplan 1995). Kaplan believes that every child has the capacity for transposition, where the parent's trauma can be undone by placing herself in the parent's position (Kaplan 1995, 225). As the parent projects her traumas through her caregiving and nurturing, the infant receives these traumas and internalizes them as part of her own existence. This is why, even if the parent never says a word, traumas may end up on the shoulders of subsequent generations.

One of the most serious harms in surviving rape is the symbolic and physical loss of control – over the situation, over the body, and essentially over life (see Herman 1992). Agency in mothering might help mothers regain this lost control. This is particularly apparent in how survivors reflect on the transmission of trauma and how cautious they are when trying – by all means possible – to prevent that transmission. This also includes the very conscious decision as to *how* and *what parts* of her war story she wants to tell and share. However, many survivors find it hard to navigate this individual agenda and personal experience together within the public and collective narrative. Although she has her own way of telling the story, children are also exposed to the collective narrative, and there is no guarantee that the mother's story will be received as more important, trustworthy, and impactful than this collective narrative. In past years of investigating survivors' attitudes to their own experiences, I have observed that survivors sometimes replace their own story with the collective narrative.

The phenomenon of trauma always takes place between individuality and collectivity (Svašek 2005), and the experiences of individual victims/survivors are always integrated into the remembrance and memory practices pursued in groups. This can function as a survival and healing strategy; dealing with a story that is not completely her own, but which is still close enough that she can relate to it, helps the survivor to move on with her own life and to survive the political and social pressures directed to her through media and the current sociopolitical milieu. At the same time, this "adopted story" has enough similarities to her own story that the woman feels connected, able to access her own pain and her very own, individualized experience. Ideally, a traumatized individual heals from the suffering caused by trauma, and in time the painful memories related to the events are forgotten. But is it the pressure of a society that contextualizes those painful events within broader sociopolitical conditions to pursue its agendas of nationalism, patriarchy, and racism? (Halbwachs 1992, 51; Zembylas 2007, 212). I wrote in my diary:

> In a way, these collective stories have been helpful for some survivors as they have done the "work" for them. As it is often important that kids "know" what happens, it is also challenging to get them to know it – through telling her own story. If the testimonies are omnipresent and accessible to the kids, she feels that all she has to do is tell her kid that she "is one of them." Yet, once she gets enough courage to do this, she is obviously ready also to tell the "rest." While some told me that it is important to tell exact details because the story should not be forgotten, others only need their kids to be supportive – for which it doesn't really matter how many details they know.
>
> (July 2018)

One of the most important factors to consider when reflecting on what mothers transmit to their offspring is an understanding of the phases of psychosocial recovery, and how mothers' openness to sharing their stories is generally related to this. Based on her clinical work with traumatized groups, Judith Herman defined three levels of recovery: (1) the establishment of safety, (2) remembrance and mourning, and (3) reconnection with ordinary life. Herman claims that traumatic events cannot be placed into a meaningful and recovered posttraumatic life if the survivor is not first able to regain her sense of safety in the new/changed environment; only once this has been established can she enter into the process of mourning and remembrance. This is the stage at which her traumatic experiences take the form of a narrated story that is heard and acknowledged by witnesses "completely, in depth and detail" (Herman 1992, 175). This includes comprehending the circumstances and context that preceded the traumatic event, and what led/allowed it to happen (Herman 1992, 176). I noticed how, for the war-rape survivors who participated in this study, these stages are subjected to various factors about which Herman does not elaborate.

Over the course of 25 years, I claim, survivors did not gradually pass from one stage to another in a hierarchical or progressive way. Instead, these phases continuously overlap, and switch places and have never truly finished. The establishment of safety in the immediate aftermath of the war, for instance, meant rebuilding houses and the community, and securing the financial and other means necessary to survive from day to day. Thus, safety (or the illusion of safety, as Herman puts it) does not necessarily reflect only the immediate postwar circumstances, where the armed conflict ends and the peace accord is officially signed. For war-rape survivors living in a divided, economically and politically unstable country and region, where many of the war crimes are continuously denied and prosecutions delayed, questions of safety remain critical in their everyday lives.

The decision to expose oneself publicly through testifying is conditioned by how much this act will increase the levels of threats and concrete risks in the everyday lives of survivors. When the survivors are mothers of underage children, the number of those willing to participate in public events related to remembrance or restorative justice processes evidently declines. Safety also has different meanings when it comes specifically to her role as a mother: one of the mothers, for instance, became concerned about safety particularly as it related to the potential sexual harassment her daughter might later experience as a teenager who would shortly commute to attend school in a nearby town.

For some mothers, the process of expressing their trauma stories – either in sharing circles with other survivors or within their families – actually helped to increase their safety. One mother explained to me how her daughters started to pay more attention to her general well-being; another told me about her son, who always made sure to give her a ride and pick her up from wherever she went, "because he tells me to do what I have to do, to get justice and put him [her perpetrator] behind bars" (Northwest Bosnia 2019). On the other hand, one survivor experienced the opposite, rather disappointing reaction: her public testimony pushed her away from what she believed was her "reconnection with ordinary life" and reintegration into the shattered postwar community:

> Since 2002 I have lived in /village/; I am alone, I lost my husband in the war. At first, I was commuting to /town/ because they had weekly gatherings, where I started to receive some psychological support and also got access to medication. But in this year, 2002, I joined this association and I did not hide it. I did not tell anyone who did not ask. I always felt they knew anyway. But after this year, I started to feel people getting more closed. I also felt a different attitude from the pharmacists; he was grumpier than before. And I think this is because I joined the association.
>
> (Northern Bosnia 2018)

Motherhood plays an important role in how survivors transit through phases of recovery proposed by Herman. There are substantial differences between those survivors who started mother-work in the immediate aftermath of the war and those who became mothers some ten years after the war, or only recently. Their own healing process, for instance, had a great impact on their way of mothering. For those who were mothers before or who became mothers right after the war, healing often takes place only when their children have become independent enough so that the mother can dedicate more time to herself. Mothers who had children right after the war were simultaneously caring for their newborns, overwhelmed by rebuilding their households, and searching for their vanished family members. Most of them sought out organized psychotherapeutic sources of support long after the war:

> I started to feel strong flashbacks right after the older one left to the /town/ to start university. And the real hell happened to me when my son got a job and

was away most of the day. It was as if the war had returned for me. I had a purpose all this time, I knew how to make myself busy for entire days. When they left, I had nothing to excuse myself.

(R57, Southeastern Bosnia 2018)

This woman stated that she only had time to immediately return to a normal life. Others agreed. Once their children were born, they focused entirely on starting a new life with them, trying to leave the war behind. Most of my interlocuters agreed that only lately had they been able to mourn publicly, acknowledging changes in the public recognition of war rapes and survivors, the shifts in public narratives, and the availability of more spaces for events that publicly remember those who vanished due to the rapes. For many, the very idea of mourning and remembering in the context of war rape is disputable: "What can I mourn? My lost virginity?" said one, and she started to laugh cynically.

You can mourn lost members of the families. We all have those who vanished, and we mourn them. But the rape? There is nothing to mourn, nor to memorialize. I wish we would remember, so we do not repeat it. But then again, how will you remember? What will you remember?

(S, Central Bosnia 2019)

Herman's notion of *reconnection with the ordinary* also demands a more in-depth understanding. For some, this happened right after the war, as they were not ready to either mourn or remember in a way that would be healthy and beneficial for their recovery. For some, mourning – which Herman defines as a separate stage – became part of what they define today as "ordinary life." Some authors (see, for instance, Kevers et al., 2016) have observed that survivors sometimes remember the period following the war more positively than their present situation. Some survivors recalled the "liveliness of the first years after Dayton" (B65, 2018), the collective aspiration in restoring social connections in the community, the hopes and dreams of social and political change that were to come, and the solidarity and cooperation. For some, it was a step toward healing; only when the times of the aftershock brought a collective need for mourning and remembrance was this healing put on hold:

I lost a lot… we all lost. But I also looked forward because all this hell was over. I remember everyone wanted to help. Because we all lost. But then years passed, and we were all waiting, but today I don't know what, what was it that we were waiting. But it got worse. We are poor today. We lost everything and we never got it back. Then we started to search for the ones we lost. And these numbers grew every day. The hope was gone, there was more and more grieving and sadness and anger instead.

(B65, 2018, Central Bosnia)

While the process of mourning, therefore, can unfold in a time sequence that differs from the one proposed by Herman, it also does not necessarily lead to healing and recovery. On the contrary, mourning can jeopardize beliefs and fantasies of a better future by exposing survivors to overwhelming amounts of pain, loss, and ongoing political denial. If mourning comes at a time that cannot be borne by the political establishment, survivors and their descendants might easily be consumed by the past. It is through the processes of mourning, says Zembylas (2007, 213), that educators (parents, family members, etc.) "will help children accept losses, subvert egoism of victimization, and become able to face more realistically their disappointments, hopes and aspirations." But what if mourning, as I believe is its current state in Bosnia-Herzegovina, becomes a vehicle for victim competition, and an arena for the eternal readiness to enter yet another conflict?

While I agree that PTSD-centered discourses and healing practices for war-rape survivors have oversimplified the individual's past, the uniqueness of one's experiences, the role of other micro- (family members) and macro- (community, state) social relations, and the institutionalized practices of remembering and mourning, open up important dimensions in the cultural and political intentionality of transmitted traumas. But again, here I am able to reflect only on those who have spoken up; those who have joined the institutionalized processes of healing – by accepting different types of support from various governmental or nongovernmental organizations, or by participating in other ways in restorative justice processes. These processes are not only regulated and mediated by different social members but are also recorded and thus become available for further analysis. But what of all the evidence that was never recorded? What of the many who might simply skip the stages – "simply," because for all the reasons one can imagine they have no access to places and practices of mourning and remembrance, either individually or collectively? What happens when mourning and remembrance happen silently, and in isolated settings? If only the completion of the first two stages might allow the survivor to reconnect with ordinary life and hence to heal from trauma, as suggested by Herman, what then happens to those who were never able to mourn?

According to Volkan, those people who are unable to mourn their losses – of their beloved, of the land, of their identities – will pass the pain of their injured selves to succeeding generations in the form of "psychological DNA" (1997, 46). The inability to mourn fuels hatred, as new generations might embrace the defense mechanisms of chosen traumas and ideologies of revenge (Volkan 2001; also, Weingarten 2003). Despite a long and rich tradition of investigating intergenerational transmission and the impacts of collective trauma, clinical and social studies have not yet found common ground as to what, how, who, and in what (trans)formations parental traumas can cause harm and destructive impacts. In contrast to clinical studies and findings of trauma transmission through DNA, most early nonclinical studies deny the existence of maladaptive behavior or psychopathological problems related to parental traumas (see for instance Bar-On et al., 1998; Danieli 1998; Sagi-Shwarz et al., 2003). For this reason, Danieli (1998) suggests shifting from the term *transmission of trauma* to *intergenerational effects of trauma*. Despite some evidence suggesting that descendants might experience similar pain or suffering, there is a great difference between the psycho-physical symptoms of survivors and cultural trauma. While understanding the psychological traumas of survivors helps us to understand the internal, individual dynamics of defense, adaptation, coping, and working-through (Tota 2006, 85), the concept of cultural trauma is more helpful when it comes to the question of how survivors narrate and share their experiences and trauma stories with their descendants.

Leading scholars in cultural memory and trauma (see Caruth 1995; Laub 1995; Felman 1995) have until now agreed about the political mediation of individual experiences into communal memory stories and have considered to be central the issue of power in the collective memory (see: Hobsbawn & Ranger 1983; Middleton & Derek 1990). This prompts me to question how much of the intergenerational effects of trauma in fact happen or are accumulated through family rearing in terms of direct transmission from survivor to child. While the survivor must cope with her own traumatic symptoms, she must also refuse the political abuse of the inflammatory potential of trauma politics run by stakeholders, religious leaders, or others whose work is centered around keeping communities divided to prevent hatred and the desire for revenge among her children. While many survivors might easily be convinced to contribute their testimonies as they believe this is crucial for the justice process, they might also easily be tricked into becoming carriers of toxic politics that have used individual traumatic experiences to form a politically driven, cautiously narrated collective trauma. Positioning the question of trauma transmission in the families takes away responsibility from the institutional and state duty to ensure the sociopolitical recovery of damaged communities. With this, the destructive emotions supposedly transmitted from traumatized individuals to their descendants an excuse for failed transitional and retributive justice processes and the institutions and political bodies that are charged with carrying them out.

This leads me to think of intentional institutional efforts in trauma transmission and how family is used as a vehicle for political agendas rather than a source of unconscious, dynamic, give-and-take behaviors, in which children are used as a captive audience (Danieli 1998, 5). Vamik Volkan (1997; 2001) applies psychoanalytic theory to explain how traumatic narratives are chosen to serve large-group identity construction. These narratives are "shared mental representations of the event, which include realistic information, fantasized expectations, intense feelings, and defenses against unacceptable thoughts" (Volkan 1997, 58). They fit a coherent story, usually one of victimization, to regain hegemonic political power in the aftermath of conflict but also to maintain its rule and its oppressive relationships over a longer period of time. Yet, the institutional use of collective memory in pursuit of present nationalistic, sexist, racist, and other oppressive ideologies on the one hand, and the role played by intergenerational trauma transmission within the family on the other, has not been sufficiently studied intersectionally and interdependently.

In the past, the intergenerational transmission of trauma effects was studied mostly in the relationship between survivor(s) and descendants, thus within the frame of intergenerational family dynamics and relationships. Danieli (1981; 1988), for instance, has even proposed "adaptational styles" of survivors' families – the victim families, the fighter families, the numb families, and the families of "those who made it" – to explain the heterogeneity in adaptation and resistance in the aftermath of traumatic events (Danieli 1981, 9). He writes that children in the survivors' families attested to "the constant psychological presence of the Holocaust at home, verbally and nonverbally, or in some cases, reported having absorbed the omnipresent experience of the Holocaust through 'osmosis'" (Danieli 1981, 5). In this sense, children of Holocaust survivors consciously (through storytelling) and unconsciously (through silences) absorbed their parents' experiences. Some internalized them as part of their identity through the images of those who vanished, and some manifested Holocaust-derived behaviors similar to those of their parents (Danieli 1981, 5). But how much of these transmissions are in fact reflections of an individual's own struggle to recover and heal? How much are they fueled by the broader political agendas of collective memory? And how many of these effects of intergenerational trauma are eventually artificially produced by the culture and the society to sustain certain patterns, ideas, and social divisions?

In our conversations, mothers did not mention that they feared transmitting symptoms such as fear, depression, lack of motivation, loss of trust, hopelessness, or powerlessness. However, among the mothers, choosing silence over sharing is seen as a way to prevent the spread of hatred toward "the Other," to prevent radical inclinations and the desire to seek revenge on "the Other," and to prevent anger and shame from entering relations with "the Other" – all to ensure that something similar will never happen again. When we talk about the transmission of trauma, we also need to talk about how trauma in the collective memory is intentionally used by governing political bodies, particularly when postconflict politics continues to profit from war-related matters and where the (post)war discourse still presents one of the most important driving forces for the current political leadership. The effects of intergenerational trauma are therefore projections similar to what Marianne Hirsch called postmemory:

> They project and reflect how children relate to the experiences of their parents, experiences that they "remember" only as the stories and images with which they grew up, but that are so powerful, so monumental, as to constitute memories in their own right.
>
> (Hirsch 1999, 8)

Unfortunately, due to the struggles that most survivors experience when sharing their experiences with their children, I was unable to collect evidence that would better explain the postmemories of children born to mothers who had been raped (but not born from rape). The few encounters that I had are rather limited, as all these children praised their mothers for their heroic and continuous fight for justice; they worshipped their mothers for their love and kindness – particularly in light of what they had been through. But what of the children whose mothers experience severe symptoms of PTSD, of mothers who were abandoned by their families, or mothers who are suicidal and severely depressed? These mothers told me how they feared that all these insuperable negative and destructive emotions would impact their children. In every group that I worked with, there were one or two who had enough courage, maturity, and openness to be able to share their stories with their children. Most of the survivors I worked with did not have this chance, yet they wanted to share their stories – not only so that the crimes would not be forgotten, but for the survivors to be relieved of their own past. Sharing their stories with their children would also mean defeating – symbolically and metaphorically – the haunting legacy, eventually allowing them to regain control over their lives by successfully integrating these stories.

A survivor who tells her story to her child brings together her personal testimony with aspects of collective memory to construct a retrospective identity, and also builds the mother-child relationship in the very moment of sharing. What is transmitted eventually shows us how, within this framework of individual/collective memory, individuals can still choose to either accept or reject their transgenerational inheritance (Thompson 2009, 15). Since Halbwachs, memory scholars have stressed that there is very little that is unique to individual, "personal" memories, as they are very soon coded in the language and subsequently enter the arena of cultural, social, and political life. Therefore, memory is navigated and navigates individuals and communities, and is a constitutional part of the everyday practices into which we are born and which we learn by doing throughout the course of our lives. They contribute significantly to group identity formations in the present, but what is more, according to Elizabeth Tonkin (1992, 111), "history is propagandist; it is to claim that people are thinking historically if they recognize themselves as part of a group and that this thought is action which helps them to be one."

While I could note that the youth with whom I have worked can "think" historically when it comes to their ethnoreligious identity, I have always wondered how they can "think" historically when it comes to the legacy of war rapes. With some of the girls who spoke with me following the workshop in 2018, I noted the victim connection and the still present threat of sexual violence. I have not been able to record any of this with the boys. The feedback they provided tended to concern the general political issue of the war, with no direct response to gender and sexuality as components of the violence. This left me with only speculative conclusions as to what children learn in their families and what might be a learning takeaway when teaching about the legacy of war rape.

Asman (2011, 31) believes that what today is packaged in the framework of "collective memory" was recognized in the 1960s and 1970s as "myths" and "ideologies." The longitude of the collective memory is therefore not limited by the moment when the survivors vanish, but with the moment when it stops serving the current societal needs and has to be changed in order to fulfill what is needed instead. This resonates with the women's fear that the war rape crimes will be forgotten as soon as they die, hence their desperate need to address the youth to ensure that it is not repeated in the future. In this type of memory, which Susan Sontag prefers to call an agreement, the community decides how certain histories must be remembered, how and why these events happened, and what accompanying (visual) materials exist to fix the story that stays in our memory (Sontag 2003, 85–86). Instead of collective memory, Sontag too thinks of ideologies which consist of connotations that impact and direct people's beliefs, feelings, and ways of thinking. Once we see the transferred collective memories as ideologies, it is perhaps easier to understand the dangers of narrated silences and the prememories of vertically and horizontally transmitted rape culture through the circles of mother–survivors.

Note

1 For more, see Močnik, Nena. 2019. Rehersing Forgiveness by Acting Out Vengeance: The Case of 'Mother of the Rapist in Embodied Research Practice with War-Rape Survivors. Research in Drama Education: The Journal of Applied Theatre and Performance 24 (4): 478–489.

Bibliography

Arendt, H. 1958. *The human condition.* Chicago: University of Chicago Press.

Arendt, H. 2003. *Responsibility and judgment.* New York: Shocken Books.

Asman, A. 2011. *Duga senka prošlosti: kultura sećanja i politika povesti.* Beograd: Biblioteka XX vek.

Bar-On, D., Eland, J., Kleber, R. J., Krell, R., Moore, Y., Sagi, A., Soriano, E., Suedfeld, P., van der Velden, P. G., and van Ijzendoorn, M. H. 1998. "Multigenerational perspectives for understanding the development sequelae of trauma across generations." *International Journal of Behavioral Development* 22: 315–338.

Barsalou, J. and Baxter, V. 2007. *The urge to remember: The role of memorials in social reconstruction and transitional justice.* Available at https://www.usip.org/publications /2007/01/urge-remember-role-memorials-social-reconstruction-and-transitional-justi ce (accessed 19 December 2019).

Booth, J. 2001. "The unforgotten: Memories of justice." *The American Political Science Review* 95(4): 777–791.

Brison, S. 2002. *Aftermath: Violence and the remaking of a self.* Princeton: Princeton University Press.

Brown, R. 2003. "Measuring individual differences in the tendency to forgive: Construct validity and links with depression." *Personality and Social Behavior Bulletin* 29 (6): 759–771.

Brudholm, T. and Grøn, A. 2011. "Picturing forgiveness after atrocity." *Studies in Christian Ethics* 24(2): 159–170.

Brudholm, T. and Rosoux, V. 2009"The unforgiving: Reflections on the resistance to forgiveness after actrocity." *Law and Contemporary Problems* 72 (33): 33–49.

Card, C. 1996. "Rape as a weapon of war." *Hypatia,* Special Issue: *Women and Violence* 11 (4): 5–18.

Card, C. 2002. *The atrocity paradigm: A theory of evil.* Oxford: Oxford University Press.

Caruth, C. 1995. *Trauma: Explorations in memory*. Baltimore, MD: JHU Press.

Cerney, M.S. 1988. ""If only …" remorse in grief therapy." *Psychotherapy Patient* 5: 235–248.

Cosgrove, L. and Konstam, V. 2008. Forgiveness and forgetting: Clinical implications for mental health counselors. *Journal of Mental Health Counseling* 30 (1): 1–13.

Danieli, Y. 1981. "Differing adaptational styles in families of survivors of the Nazi Holocaust." *Child Today* 10 (5): 6–10.

Danieli, Y. 1998. "Introduction: History and conceptual foundations." In Y. Danieli (Ed.), *International handbook of multigenerational legacies of trauma* (1–17). New York: Plenum Press.

Derrida, J. 2000. "On forgiveness." *Studies in Practical Philosophy* 2 (2): 81–102.

Felman, S. 1995. *Testimony: Crises of witnessing in literature, psychoanalysis and history*. New York: Routledge.

Halbwachs, M. 1992. *On collective memory*. Chicago, IL: University of Chicago Press.

Herman, J. 1992. *Trauma and recovery. The aftermath of violence – From domestic abuse to political terror*. New York: Basic Books.

Hirsch, M. 1999. "Projected memory: Holocaust photographs in personal and public fantasy." In M. Bal, J. V. Crewe, and L. Spitzer (Eds.), *Acts of memory: Cultural recall in the present* (3–23). New Hampshire, New England: University Press of New England.

Hobsbawn, E. and Ranger, T. 1983. *The invention of tradition*. Cambridge: Cambridge University Press.

Holmgren, M. R. 1993. "Forgiveness and the intrinsic value of persons." *American Philosophical Quarterly* 30 (4): 341–352.

Kaplan, L. J. 1995. *No voice is ever wholly lost: An explorations of the everlasting attachment between parent and child*. New York: Simon & Schuster.

Kolnai, A. 1973. "Forgiveness." *Proceedings of the Aristotelian Society* 74 (91): 106.

Kristeva, J. and Rice, A. 2002. "Forgiveness: An interview." *PMLA* 117 (2): 278–295.

Laub, D. 1995. "Truth Sand testimony: The process and the struggle." In C. Caruth (Ed.), *Trauma: Explorations in memory* (45–61). Baltimore, MD: JHU Press.

Looney, A. T. 2015. *Vladimir Jankélévitch: The time of forgiveness*. New York: Fordham University Press.

May Schott, R. 2004. "The atrocity paradigm and the concept of forgiveness." *Hypatia: A Journal of Feminist Philosophy* 19 (4): 204–211.

Mendelhoff, D. 2009. "Trauma and vengeance: Assessing the psychological and emotional effects of post-conflict justice." *Human Rights Quarterly* 31 (3): 592–623.

Middleton, D. and Derek, E. 1990. *Inquiries in social construction. Collective remembering*. Thousand Oaks, CA: Sage Publications.

Minow, M. 1998. *Between vengeance and forgiveness: Facing history after genocide and mass violence*. Boston: Beacon Press.

Ricoeur, P. 1973. *Memory, history, forgetting*. Chicago: University of Chicago Press.

Thompson, L. Y., Snyder, C. R., Hoffman, L., Michael, S. T., Rasmussen, H. N., Billings, L. S., Heinze, L., Neufeld, J. E., Shorey, H. S., Roberts, J. C., and Roberts, D. E. 2005. "Dispositional forgiveness of self, others, and situations." *Journal of Personality* 73 (2): 313–359.

Thompson, P. 2009. "Family myth, models, and denials in the shaping of individual life paths." In P. Thompson and D. Bertaux (Eds.), *Between generations: Family models, myths and memories* (13–38). London: Transaction Publishers.

Tonkin, E. 1992. *Narrating our pasts: The social construction of oral history*. Cambridge: Cambridge University Press.

Tota, A. L. 2006. Public memory and cultural trauma. *The Public* 13 (3): 81–94.

Sagi-Schwartz, A., van Ijzendoorn, M., Grossmann, K. E., Grossmann, K., and Koren-Karie, N. 2003. "Attachment and traumatic stress in female holocaust child survivors and their children." *American Journal of Psychiatry* 160: 1086–1092.

Sontag, S. 2003. *Regarding the pain of others*. New York: Picador.

Svašek, M. 2005. "The politics of chosen trauma: Expellee memories, emotions and identities." In K.E. Milton and M. Svašek (Eds.), *Mixed emotions: Anthropological studies of feeling* (195–214). Oxford: Berg.

van der Veer, G. 1998. *Counselling and therapy with refugees and victims of trauma: Psychological problems of victims of war, torture and repression*. New Jersey: Wiley.

Volkan, V.D. 1997. "Transgenerational transmissions and chosen traumas: An aspect of large-group identity." *Group Analysis* 34(1): 79–97.

Volkan, V. D. 2001. "Transgenerational transmissions and chosen traumas: An aspect of large-group identity." *Group Analysis* 34 (1): 79–97.

Webb, J. R., Bumgarner, D. J., Conway-Williams, E., Dangel, T., and Hall, B. B. 2017. "A consensus definition of self-forgiveness: Implications for assessment and treatment." *Spirituality in Clinical Practice* 4 (3): 216–227.

Weingarten, K. 2003. *Common shock: Witnessing violence every day: How we are harmed, how we can heal*. New York: Dutton Books.

Zembylas, M. 2007. "The politics of trauma: Empathy, reconciliation and education." *Journal of Peace Education* 4(2): 207–224.

6 War-rape legacies

Transmission, agency, transformation

Toward the changing paradigms in healing from trauma: Sociotherapy and trauma of war rape as social responsibility

Today's postwar generation has embraced the legacy of rape in their own manner, taking ownership as community members, and they have their own ways of approaching and dealing with it. As I discussed in previous chapters, the culture of silence and the way stigma was attached to survivors but is only lately discussed from a societal viewpoint created the postwar rehabilitation process that is centered around individual (psycho)approaches to trauma healing rather than using collective (socio)therapy. Only when responsibility for historical events is shared among all of society's members can we transform the culture of impunity into a culture of accountability. An person-centered approach to trauma among war-rape survivors is perhaps the reason why the legacy of war rape is seen through the prism of one's medical condition rather than as a sociopolitical issue that should occupy the same place in peace education as working on interethnic and inter-religious dialogue. The legacy of war rape and its related stigma are about *healing* rather than *educating*, *rehabilitation* rather than *prevention*, *abolishment* rather that *transformation*. To prevent the negative effects of trauma transmission from mother–survivors of war rape, I propose to include the legacy of war rape in education, in formats of prevention that would allow for the transformation of continued toxic narratives, patterns, behaviors, and politics of violent sexualities.

While scholars widely understand rape-related stigma through the structures of patriarchy and/or gender and sexuality, rape stigma in the context of war should also be understood along narrow political lines. In relation to the broader notions of political power, governance, and domination, the stigma that keeps survivors silent also serves to obstruct the restorative and retributive justice processes while preventing survivors from offering evidential testimonies about the crimes. The estimated number of women raped during the war in Bosnia-Herzegovina varies from 20,000 to 50,000. Less than 1 percent of this number have been officially registered; the vast majority have never spoken out. A stigma-free society where 20,000 survivors are able to provide evidence without being socially punished or living in fear or insecurity would prevent their rapists from denying their crimes and escaping prosecution. Therefore, part of the stigmatization perpetuated by relatives (e.g., husbands, fathers, brothers, or sons) might be understood through the feminist lens of patriarchy. Sometimes, the same men who shame and punish women through abuse and abandonment project their own personal traumas and, in some cases, their own guilt and responsibility. In as much as we focus our attention only on "victims" (or "survivors"), our massive knowledge gap concerning the perpetrators precludes an understanding of most of the sociopolitical dynamics, including stigmatization, and merely slows the prosecution of perpetrators. Working with stigma without stigma power further perpetuates the culture of impunity. What we wonder is whether full recovery, healing, and closure for women survivors is at all possible when certain aspects of restorative justice have not yet been achieved.

One of the factors that contributes to the perpetuation of both silence and stigma is therefore the individualized treatment of traumatic experiences, in which the focus is on the survivor and her own ability to heal. I wonder to what extent breaking the silence of war rape actually contributes to reconciliation and what its role in peace education or general peacebuilding might be. While it is evident that breaking the silence is important in terms of transitional justice and punishment, it is not necessarily crucial in trauma transmission prevention. My diary after a workshop with a group of teenagers reads as follows:

> I was posing different sorts of questions, of course being careful about the language and potential triggers. However, they would not respond to anything. They just look – not even to me, but away. / ... name ... / was mumbling something, just because it's how he always is – he always has to say something. But at this moment, I could not really grasp what he was about to say. As he was always early for the class, I invited him today and asked him directly if the group felt uncomfortable or why they were silent. He said it's not about being uncomfortable but being tired of talking about something that is not "theirs." He said, "I don't know what to tell you, except that these stories are bad."

When thinking how to position the legacy of war rapes in today's peace education and broader reconciliation efforts, it is crucial to understand the contribution of social actors in stigmatization and how this prevents approaching the topic with the aim of working with the survivors and descendants in a constructive way. Elsewhere in the book, I mentioned a testimony from a mother who was initially abandoned and left behind by her three adult kids when, in 1996, she disclosed her experiences. But today, she has reestablished and normalized her relationships with them and her grandchildren. In correspondence, she shared that since their return, they have never again broached this topic (despite the fact that she would like to), yet today, she understands their reaction as an impulsive response and even shock (field notes, Northeast Bosnia, 2018). She has been *working through* the traumatic symptoms like depression, physical pain, and anxiety, as well as self-stigmatization as a consequence of being abandoned. Today, she claims she has come to terms with what happened to her; she feels safe and empowered among other survivors in the organization that she joined in 2015. Her kids have also *worked through* and come to the point of being able to return to her and, therefore, accept her *as she is today* – if not also her past war-rape experience. This case helps us understand that a focus on individual work with trauma is not sufficient when it comes to stigma and that, in future work with survivors, engaging family members from the beginning is key to a more inclusive and integrated rehabilitation practice in the aftermath of a conflict. Also, when collecting evidence about the stigmatization and ostracism of war-rape survivors, we tend to ignore the long-term dynamics and the attitudes and relationships that eventually change over the course of years. In order to more fully approach rehabilitation and integration in the aftermath of a conflict, and also to take into consideration all the risks of transmitting traumatic legacies, I therefore see the necessity for the traumatized individuals being contextualized, located in their environment and, most importantly, within their everyday social interactions (Akman 2015, 10). Centering the medical symptoms, survivors' social status, and perspective on mental health as the consequences of different social factors rather than intra- or individual psychological battles is often insignificant in this field.

On several occasions, I engaged youngsters in conversation, asking if it is important to talk about sexual violence – in war and peace – and about its consequences and impacts. Easy access to knowledge and information (mostly thanks to the tools of information technology) has resulted in today's generation dealing very differently with sexuality – despite being raised in a patriarchal heteronormative context, for instance – and it remains questionable whether there is, in fact, anything we can learn from the history of violent sexuality. Another phenomenon, which I called *narrated silences*, accompanies any consideration of teaching sexuality and trauma transmission. The reproduction and use of narrated silences is of particular interest to survivors but can have damaging effects on youth.

In recent years, one could see an increased interest in engaging in some type of sociotherapy and antistigmatization work regarding war-rape legacies in Bosnia-Herzegovina. In addition to direct campaigns and activism primarily initiated and performed by survivors, their supporters, and (health) community centers (for activism and feminist agency see Helms 2014), different members of society have employed the theme of war rapes and legacies in documentaries, journalistic portraits, and artistic depictions in literature, film, theater, and painting. These often politically motivated productions have been generally considered as action toward symbolic reparation (Simić & Volčić 2014) and artistic memory work (Asavei 2019, 2). More or less well recognized yet not always well received across the region of the Western Balkans are *As If I Am Not There*, a novel by Slavenka Drakulić (1999); *Grbavica*, a film by Jasmila Žbanić (2006), and *In the Land of Blood and Honey* (2011), a movie by Angelina Jolie. Each has put the crime of war rape and stories of survivors from Bosnia-Herzegovina on the global map. The mission of this "artistic memory work" is giving voice to the crimes, with the stories based on real events and testimonies but represented through the subjective interpretation of the creators, with fictional settings and imagined characters. Even though the authors never claimed originality or authenticity in their stories, media wars about misleading appropriation and survivors' resentment has become kind of the traditional response to anyone but survivors narrating their stories. The anger and frustration that survivors express when witnessing their stories being represented and (mis)interpreted are correlated with Mieke Bal's argument.

> Rape cannot be visualized because the experience is, physically as well as psychologically, *inner*. /.../ In this sense, rape is by definition imagined; it can only exist as experience and as memory, as *image* translated into signs, never adequately objectifiable.
>
> (Bal 2001, 100)

Reenactments of war rapes and, more generally, war in Bosnia-Herzegovinahave sparked several studies (Helms 2014; Simić & Volčić 2014; Lengel 2018) examining the potential risk of performativity as a vehicle for social change in sociopolitical contexts where such representations and "voicing" can in fact risk retraumatization, marginalization, and the further deepening of the stigmatization of survivors (Solga 2006; Thaler 2018, 77). Reenacting war rape can be described as

> a double-edged sword: it both "solves" the problem of rape – it cannot be prosecuted if it is not known, and it cannot be known if the victim refuses to raise the hue and cry. /.../ Made a spectacle, turned into theater, rape slips away from the woman it haunts as its inner, invisible effects effectively disappear.
>
> (Solga 2006, 61)

To this inner, unspeakable experience, the reenactment therefore always risks being narratively and visually insufficient and painful to witness – especially for survivors. It is almost impossible for the audience to see and understand survivors' original trauma through a "standardized version of her suffering" (Solga 2006, 61), which extends survivor pain in representing what is arguably an "inaccessible event" (Solga 2006, 57). For the audience as witness, the rape representation furthermore navigates moral instruction in understanding *the pain of the aftermath*. Conveyed through the narratives of silence and shame, war-rape reenacts recreate the images that help to enhance stigmatization of war-rape survivors.

This strong *artistic* component also characterizes the four performances produced by UNFPA, *Ta Tvoja Mund Harmonika* (2016); *Sjenka Duše* (2016); *Mi Smo Preostali* (2017), and *Žute Čizme* (2018) that use the elements of expressive and physical theater to invite postwar youth, survivors, and local audiences into active dialogue and campaigning against stigma for the better reintegration into society of survivors of sexual violence. Performances have been realized as the outcome of the applied drama training and scripts, and the dramaturgical concepts were based on research previously conducted by UNFPA in the frame of the project *Seeking Care, Support, and Justice for Survivors of Conflict Related Sexual*

Violence in BiH (2015).[1] One of the project outcomes was also the previously mentioned research. The idea of using theater was not to traumatize the audience, nor for sharing the testimonies of survivors; rather, the performances aimed to open up discussion on the "role of the society and individuals in stigmatization" (Farmer 2018) and to enhance emphatic attitudes toward survivors (Osmić 2018). The creators strove to look at the consequences of war rapes today and here, particularly from the perspective of the relationship between society and survivors (from this direction).

In this way, it is also understandable why the direct involvement of survivors and their responses were not given priority. Osmić explains that performance emphasizes empathy, support, and solidarity to encourage audiences to think and discuss the topic from today's perspective rather than retraumatizing and bringing back memories from the past. The mission of those performances is hence not only informative, but also educational, or *transformative*. This was clear with the original choices of the format of forum theater, which essentially is a theater that aims to open up and engage in dialogue with the audience with the very deliberate goal of seeking solutions for the problems being staged. However, during the process, it became clear that fighting against stigma is far more conceptual than can be simplified in a performative statement and asking the audience to provide the answer. In conversation with Marija Farmer, she confirmed that the audience are also usually members of society who are not in need of having their prejudices and stereotypes changed. The very decision to spend an evening witnessing a performance about war-related rapes and stigmatization can already be read as active participation in fighting against stigma. Theater with an audience that is eager to witness and engage, even if only through being physically present with their bodies, could use those bodies to strengthen awareness about the topic's importance and to have the topic penetrate deeper into the realms of social narratives, present ideologies, and policies. It co-creates social conditions that are safe and open enough to embrace the most challenging procedures of retributive and restorative justice that need to be responded to for society as a whole to heal.

With intentional goals in dialogical theater, those performances in a (perhaps less intentional) way also pave transitional paths from individualistic (psychotherapeutic) to more systematic and structural visions of dealing with the stigma of war-rape survivors. Those performances function as an important mediator in these yet to be developed forms of sociotherapy, which includes demands for social members to change (not only survivors) and promote the importance of change on a wider scale. However, they do not instruct us much about the power structures and the symbolic power behind the (political) motives, in particular, for keeping those women stigmatized. Apparently one reason can be found in historically embedded structures of patriarchy, and this can be simplified through the examples of women being abandoned or shamed for their sexuality in their own families. But I want to speculate further by opening the arena to the fact that those male family members of female rape survivors who stayed in the country during the war were dragged into the complex war machinery as also victims/ survivors, witnesses, or for some of them, as perpetrators. This complexity in the variety of war experiences, if looked at from the wider family, top-down perspective, occurred to me in my work with survivors whose spouses were recruited as camp guards or spent their inter-war time in places that are today well-known for different forms of atrocities and violence against local inhabitants.

During my field work in 2018, I encountered three examples where my focus was initially on women survivors and their traumatic stories, but where we experienced difficulties in continuing the collaboration when I started to collect (too much) information about their spouse and the spouse's activities during the war. When trying to understand the survivors within this complex nexus of family relationships and intersectional/conflictual legacies from the war that each family member can have, one needs to assess the motives of stigmatization also from the position of (symbolic) power and any restorative/retributive justice that such an assessment could shatter. Yet the power structures that lead family members to abandon women survivors are not necessarily only of a patriarchal background. What if the stigmatization is a mechanism that helps some individuals get away with the crimes; to preserve impunity and denial and to slow down any legal procedures in prosecuting war crimes and achieving restorative justice.

In the previously mentioned UNFPA research with 1,000 random respondents by phone, the investigators concluded that only about 3 percent of the respondents had negative attitudes toward survivors. In other words, they blamed the persons to be blamed; they believed that they deserved it because they provoked it and that it could have been prevented (UNFPA 2015, 15). Very similarly, the positive, engaged, compassionate response has been reported from the above-mentioned performances that were staged in three different cities (Sarajevo, Banja Luka, and Prijedor); hence, in a different context and an audience with different war experiences. However, how do we fill the gap between the survivors' claims of being stigmatized, on the one hand, and the research data and audience's positive, nonstigmatizing or antistigmatizing response, on the other hand? Farmer (in interview 2019) explained that she is aware that the young people who participated in the training and the audience and witnessed the performances were obviously selected. However, this population represents "80% of those that we call the 'silent majority'" (in interview 2019), and hence, they are the target group that can noticeably contribute to breaking the stigma.

> You are actually not working directly with the bullies, this is ... they just need to be jailed ... you can't raise awareness among those, there is no dialogue, this needs to be punished, and regulated with the law. These people, they can be involved in different types of psychological social support. This means that you work with the silent majority, with those that pretend not to see what is wrong, because if they join the activists, they can be exposed and subjected to the violence, to this cycle of violence, but if they keep silent, they actually join the bullies with this. They, from one side, say this does not concern me, I have nothing against /this population/, therefore I do not intervene. But from the other side, if you do not intervene, you actually allow bullies to perpetuate the violence. And of course, there is always the paranoia of engaging,

that you will expose yourself to the same type of stigmatization, violence, or otherwise.

(Farmer in an interview, 2019)

With another example, Farmer proposed that direct violence emerging from or based on stigmatization be regulated by law and violators immediately prosecuted. The next step toward psychosocial healing of survivors would involve the evidence that would facilitate a direct connection between stigmatization and silencing and those accountable for crimes but who have not yet been prosecuted. Because if women remain silent, the crimes go unprosecuted; society acts with impunity. When women do not speak, mechanisms with shattering social repercussions must be employed. Stigmatization that leads to shaming and ostracism is working in circumstance.

The responsibility for healing that is for now imposed on survivors through an individual approach to psychotherapy has been shared by the members of the silent majority, and it is only a natural development of this psychosocial healing to start approaching systematic and structural foundations that keep certain social members stigmatized and discriminated against. To deal with powerful political bodies, particularly in a corrupt, unstable, divided, and fragile country such as postconflict Bosnia-Herzegovina, is of course the most challenging part of healing; for some, it is even risky and dangerous. But without considering stigma power in antistigmatization projects is to focus on stigma as a political apparatus that enables "the structures, mechanisms, and justifications of power to function" (Foucault 2008, 85) and will hardly push the entire process of healing forward.

However, while they are investing time, energy, and sometimes money in their individual healing, much less is being changed in terms of structures. When I asked the participants in my research how the ideal closure of healed trauma would look, one burst out, "To prosecute those who freely walk in these very streets everyday" (Central Bosnia 2018). The impact of initiatives that I listed above as examples of engaged social environment is therefore crucial not only in terms of retributive justice in the form of artistic memory work but is, moreover, paving a pathway to justice in the prevention of sexual violence in current and future conflicts.

Working with stigma power emphasizes developing systematic mechanisms that empower survivors to speak up by building alliances between citizens and important social (and religious) institutions. The inclusion of a criminal investigation element is crucial as it is one of the most important promotors of impunity and stigma and is often reported to be used by individuals in power who are part of the criminal justice system. If there is no aim to consider stigmatization of war-related rape survivors in multifaceted responses that include the criminal justice system, at least over the long run, such interventions will ultimately fail to break the stigma. Overestimating the role of individual society members in working with the stigma concept and simultaneously under-addressing the stigma power enforces the rape myths and ignores the necessity for fundamental changes of rape culture – both in war and during peace. Narrowly conceived interventions that

include very specific and limited social circles and do not penetrate those that foster both discursive and physical obstacles to prosecuting the crimes of war rapes
keeps the issue of the war-rape legacy on the margins of the political agenda.

While emphasizing the importance of random society members, the supporters
of integrating war-rape survivors into society are important for easing the survivors' everyday lives. Stigma power can only be broken and healing improved if
the individuals in question are no longer just random citizens (like in the survey
by UNFPA or the audience members) but rather are the structure(s) behind the
actions that create stigmatization and distribute the ideas, prejudices, and beliefs
that prefer survivors in the position of silenced victim. In the end, what does
research that provides perceptions of war-rape survivors by randomly chosen
individuals, with little or nothing else known of their identities (gender, social
class, geographic location such as rural or urban setting, age, and their direct/
indirect involvement/connection to the war) contribute to our knowledge of the
mechanisms of stigmatization? I claim that only by fully understanding how those
individuals are embedded in the broader political structures can one understand
the motives for stigmatization of survivors. As an illustration, I would like to
provide another example from my field research work with a female survivor
whose two male family members had been mobilized to the front lines and had
therefore actively participated in combat – whether they committed any crimes
is impossible to learn from my conversation with this woman. The survivor feels
stigmatized by these same two family members – being looked down on, having
blame for the rape thrown in her face, being insulted as *nisam vrijedna* (I am not
worthy) – and hence, she is not an isolated case, and these two members of her
family are not "random" members of society. Therefore, stigmatized survivors,
with all their pain, labels, struggles, and traumatic legacies are surrounded by
members of society (family, friends, work colleagues) who survived war as well
– as survivors of violence, witnesses, or perpetrators.

In order to study, analyze, and envision how mother–survivors might be better
included in existing peace education and peace building programs, I first wanted
to draft a model of the psychosocial healing process of survivors (see Figure 6.1).

This model, the stages of which are in the form of concentric circles, emphasizes how healing and social recovery includes and targets different members of
society, both inside and outside of a survivor's family circles. This model proposes the act of "disclosure" as central to initiating the entire process of destigma-
tization and to integrating the traumatic experiences of survivors into a broader
social (history) script. At the circle, the supporting mechanisms emphasize the
importance of survivors speaking out in order to break the stigma. In this way,
the success of social rehabilitation and antistigmatization is perceived through the
survivor's individual strength of disclosure.

Arguing in the second section of this text that for the last two decades, most of
the focus was given to disclosure, I discussed how the recent increased production of community theater performances and the consequential visibility and recognition of the survivors' statuses clearly marked a transition toward the second
circle of enclosure. At the second level, some type of social participation must

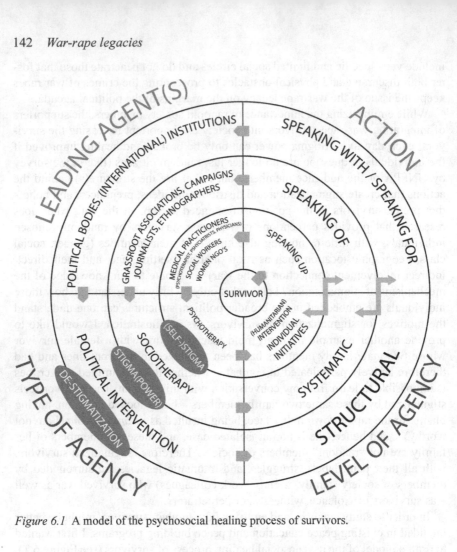

Figure 6.1 A model of the psychosocial healing process of survivors.

be present to start the act of accepting the survivor's story. At this stage, society-oriented projects that use and appropriate testimonies work together with the survivors as some type of social agent/agency responsible for breaking the stigma. The main goal of those initiatives is (re)integration, and therefore, the enclosure of survivors' experiences and present social roles and statuses to other postwar reconciliation, peace building, resilience, and healing processes. The performances mentioned here are examples of social actions that enhance the enclosure. In contrast to the first level, the agency here comes from the top down, meaning that it includes institutions and social actors with symbolic power – in education (school, nonformal programs), the arts, or the developmental and humanitarian sectors. The objectives of those actions do not necessarily target those directly involved in crimes or justice processes related to them. Rather, they seek to show support, "to just be there as human," and for survivors, this is sometimes already quite a lot (Farmer 2018). Embracing the topic from the position of "this is our story, too" (Farmer 2019), the social environment where survivors live encloses their experiences and testimonies and accepts them as components of current sociopolitical affairs. While many disclosure activities were performed ad hoc and as learning-by-doing projects, enclosure became more systematic, entering the sphere of structural agency. This phase differs from disclosure because what is in focus is not the women's stories but stories of tellers:

> We deal with the soul that says: I see you, I hear you. /.../ I am here, I am showing the support, and this is what I can do as individual at this moment /.../ I am on the side of humanity, I do not know yet how to help, but together, we will find a way.
>
> (Farmer 2019)

The goal is no longer speaking up by survivors to disclose, to put the crimes on display; neither is it "speaking for" by supporters, as in the artistic memory work. Rather, these performances are on a mission of "speaking of" – not of them but of us – of our perceptions, support in stigmatization through an "it does not concern me" attitude, and of actions to be taken while everyone waits for the structural changes. While scholars understand rape-related stigma primarily through the structures of patriarchy and/or gender and sexuality, rape stigma in the context of war should also be understood in narrow political terms. In relation to broader notions of political power, governance, and domination, a stigma that keeps survivors silent also serves to slow down the restorative and retributive justice processes, while preventing the survivors from providing evidence for crimes in the form of their testimonies.

As is clearly illustrated in the diagram, working with the stigma attached to war-rape survivors over the long term only invites other social members to actively contribute to the antistigmatization processes in the later stages. While I support the idea of the importance of survivors' voices, I also think that the legacy of war rapes or any other collective atrocities does not concern only survivors. If we believe that collective memory is created to direct the social dynamics of future generations, then those generations have to have a voice. The work challenging the stigma of survivors is still mainly to be found in the domain of survivors themselves and in organizations that deal with gender and women's issues. In a way, this supports the social perception that gender-based violence is a women's issue, and the stigma of sexual violence is one from the survivors. I believe that knowledge and information collected from mothers who are survivors must be incorporated more broadly in peace programs and must address young people cross-generationally, cross-ethnically, cross-religiously, cross-gender, and beyond.

Transmitted traumas, chosen memories

To start the conversation on what a mother transmits to her children, either in the form of values and beliefs or in the form of conscious or unconscious learning processes and socialization, I first asked a group of survivors to reflect on their childhood and how they remembered their own mothers. Asking them to write down the memories and associations with their mothers was an emotional exercise. Among other items, the following associations appeared on almost every sticky note:

worth/courageous/strong/empathic/mild/wise/
good housewife/heroine/clean/warm/understanding/
supportive/my best friend

Together we looked at what they had written down. There was not a single negative memory. There were no indicators that their mothers had mothered in oppressive, sometimes physically violent patriarchal families. Indeed, they associated their mothers with self-sacrificing love and tenderness and a metaphorical safe space; and they saw themselves as being the same. Afterward, I asked them to write down the associations and characteristics that they wish their own children would write on the sticky notes. They wrote the same, adding "only what I got from my mother, that is love and grace" (R63, Brčko 2018). They want their children to see them as courageous, and as role models with moral and ethical values. Although aware of their own trauma, and that it can be transmitted, most agreed that they work very hard to block the transmission of shame and guilt related to their war-rape experiences. Some specifically mentioned the struggle that they experience in regard to the female body, the hatred related to the memory of the abuse and how, with this in mind, they want their daughters to love their bodies.

Most worry about the mark that their trauma might leave on their children; to a certain extent, they confirmed how "the child suckles 'the black milk' of trauma, relishes and absorbs it, cultivates its bitter taste, as if it were a vital substance, as if it were existence itself" (in Kaplan 1996, 224). Manheim claims that individuals between the ages of 12-25 are particularly prone to use their life experiences during this period to determine their entire personal development. In addition, each person is to a certain extent labeled by the characteristics of the specific historical/generational period in which she lives, which affects her attitudes, beliefs, habits, perceptions, interpretations of the world, and cultural matrix. According to Manheim, this means that, despite individual memory and the trauma-infused 'milk' that a child consumes from her mother, this memory can still be erased by the broader generational memory.

In his text, *International Aspects of the Conflict in the Former Yugoslavia* (1998), Eduard Klein claims that breaking the intergenerational transmission of "negative emotions" that derive from the unresolved injustices of the past is only possible when the patriarchal family transforms into a modern one, in which family upbringing does not rely on the absolute, untouchable authority of the father's power. With respect to the events in the former Yugoslavia, Klein seeks to blame the authoritarian education that encourages the development of divisive projections and the creation of the enemy and identification with authoritarian figures (Klein 1998, 291). Although in decline, he notes the frequent and dangerous motivations assigned to children by their parents, "primarily mothers" (Klein 1998, 293), to avenge those who vanished during the war. Klein situates such vengeful behavior in the pathological family dynamics of the people in the anthropological and geographical "South," namely the Balkans, but also in Northern Africa and Latin America. In such societies, he writes, mothers are responsible for the transmission of cultural models, values, and emotions.

The wounded mother, whose husband was killed, is therefore the first to "wake up her son every morning with the words: 'Go and kill the murderers of your father'" (Klein 1998, 293). In this vein, he ignores what Manheim (1952) confirmed before him: that trauma transmission is a two-way process, in which the older generation, with its strengthened social dynamics, becomes receptive to the ideas of the young. On the contrary, Klein assigns to the mothers full responsibility for nurturing hatred, while at the same time acknowledging that mothers can also break the chain of vengeance and thus the transmission of destructive social behaviors. Yet the psychosocial support offered to war-rape survivors in dealing with their trauma, for instance, has not really anticipated including both parents and children in these processes; there is no platform where children and parents can speak, express, and embrace their feelings and war-related suffering. This would help to relieve the pathological emotions that are now transmitted and later incorporated in the aftermath of war into new forms of structural and direct violence (Klein 1998, 294).

Das suggests that, to avoid the negative emotions of the past in everyday life, the violent past must be processed, and places for processing, working through, and integrating the collected traumas must be established (Das 2007, 20). It is therefore not necessarily the emotions of rage, hatred, and vengeance that can plunge a society into "debilitating paralysis" (Das, ibid.) but a lack of places and opportunities to mourn. Storytelling, sharing experiences between generations, and bearing witness are crucial practices for processing the past; however, to allow this to happen, safe spaces for sharing must first be created.

Survivors realize how important it is that their stories are told, not only to make their own pasts comprehensible to themselves, but to help them create new identities in the aftermath of the war and in the memory culture. For a social researcher in the context of transmitted collective traumas, these stories are important because they tell us how violent experiences are remembered and how the information from remembered experiences is selected – what is told and what is omitted. While some survivors took as their life mission testifying to ensure that all war crimes were prosecuted, others believed that leaving their pasts behind and committing fully to their families would help them to forget and to reestablish what they thought would be normal and balanced lives. Telling one's story is a fearful experience not only because every new account will make it harder to forget, but because re-telling it involves reliving it, or experiencing it again (Schank 1990, 116).

Over time, the individual stories of survivors have changed, sometimes due to the availability of new evidence, sometimes because survivors have managed to put the shattered pieces into a more coherent wholeness and, in many cases, because the story needed to be adjusted to serve the needs of restorative justice processes. Despite the uniqueness of every single experience among the survivors, sharing circles helped them to build a story that is simultaneously owned by everyone, in part because "only a woman who experienced the same as I did, can understand me" (S62, Central Bosnia 2015) and partly because those sharing circles are for some women the only places where they can be survivors of war rape. In other contexts – in their communities, and particularly in their families – openly sharing what they survived could mean losing their loved ones or being abandoned. When asked if they want to share their testimony with their children or grandchildren, most survivors answered positively. When I asked what holds them back, one survivor explains:

> Let M /the woman who sits across the circle/ tell you what happened with her three daughters when she told them! She sent them away during the war, and she for sure spared what happened to her from also happening to her daughters! But now that she told them, they shame her and tell her she lies. I would rather keep my mouth shut and bring this with me to my grave than allow my kids to abandon me this way. It is hard for me to live with this secret and every day I think, what if they know anyway? And any moment I feel, now is the time, believe me, I think of this every day. But I just never do it. I cannot know for sure how they will react, and it is better to say nothing.
>
> (M64, Brčko 2018)

Generally, the survivors mention three reasons as to why they felt the need to share their experiences. First, many of them believe that doing so would help them with their recovery and would bring relief to their family life. However, as some of them had been abandoned or shamed by family members, most could not trust that their family was ready to hear. While carrying the burden of trauma is heavy, even the small chance that their children would react negatively was not worth the risk. Second, they feel that they are losing strength and the persistence necessary to continue the fight against denial and for their rights as they relate to reparations. They are getting older and changes in this regard are small and slow in coming. They believe that their children are better equipped with this knowledge and digitally connected not only locally but internationally and that they could be more successful in achieving the rights of survivors. Third, they believe that informing and familiarizing their children with what happened to them will put an end to the cycles of violence and prevent a repeat of similar histories with their own children.

Working interchangeably between the two generations, I have noticed a tension between *memorialization fatigue* on the one side and *persistent silence* on the other: while many survivors fight daily to break the silence that perpetuates impunity and in this way achieve justice, the postwar generations, today's teenagers, often feel overloaded by the war memories that overshadow the problems of their own *zeitgeist*, such as unemployment and mass depopulation. Moreover, while survivors express their worries and concerns about transmitting their own traumas, they also want to be able to control and prevent this from happening again, because "what happened to us should never be forgotten" (M, Sarajevo 2018). In a way, the socially imposed, postconflict necessity of always remembering uses the new generations as sort of "remembrance vehicle" to carry the burden of remembrance of the violent events and atrocities of past generations. While many survivors actively create and reproduce the collective memory, their work with youth made me question if the same memory practices used by survivors might serve the postwar youth – or should every generation create its own approach to the survivors' memory practices and create its own memory? – in a way that *they* want or need to remember. What then is the legacy that survivors want to leave consciously and with anticipated goals and purposes for future generations? What aspects of the war rapes should be remembered, and which should be set aside as too dangerous?

Most mothers are conscious of their trauma and the effects that it can have on their families. They choose to avoid speaking about the war in their homes primarily to protect their children from the pain and to not burden themselves with a history that is not theirs:

> I know that my son would be in pain if I just mentioned to him what happened to me. Sometimes I think he would be angry and maybe he would want to attack this man who did this to me. But to me it is more unbearable to imagine how much pain he would feel to think about this. I think he feels my love and how kind I am to him and that I would give everything for him. I think he would suffer a lot knowing how much I suffered. But I don't want him to suffer. This is my pain, not his. He deserves a good life, without this pain, and I will give it to him.
>
> (J54, North East Bosnia 2018)

Navigating the memory between the desire to share in order to remember and the will to protect their children from potentially traumatic repercussions is as important for survivors as the other levels of their individual and collective healing. The transgenerational family culture, says Thompson (in Bertaux & Thompson 2005, 15) shows how "within that framework individuals can choose not only to accept but also to reject their transgenerational inheritance." Life stories, read as true or mythical, are a form of transmission, impacting social histories and building up individual and collective identities and memories (Bertaux & Thompson, ibid.). The fear that survivors express about their children's reactions when getting to know their stories shows that they understand the transmission of trauma as a dialogical process in which the new generation is not simply a passive receiver of life stories. In the same way, while mothers are very cautious about what they transmit from their traumatic experiences, at the same time they transmit certain inherited cultural patterns about which they have never really reflected. In this vein, for instance, the normalized and accepted aspects of domestic violence are often not considered as being related to war rape.

For the stories to be told to future generations, the process demands self-analysis (*who am I as a mother–survivor?*) and an active approach to identity construction (*who do I want to be for my children?*). These two contrasting identities are very often in conflict as mothers struggle with how to be survivors while at the same time avoiding the stigmatizing representations with which this identity is usually associated. Many fear that the stigma of sexual violence will prevail over their mothering:

> First I am mother to my kid. I have survived rape, but this is not important for her. I want her to see me as a mother, not as a survivor. But I would also like to tell her what I survived. If I could only tell her without her seeing me as a survivor, this would be the best for me.
>
> (A60, Central Bosnia 2018)

To protect their children from trauma transmission, mother–survivors report that they intentionally avoid speaking about this at home. This is similar to Veena Das's observation in her *Life and Words* (2007) that a dissociation, a form of psychic splitting, has been used by survivors who had to care for their children and families both in the catastrophic circumstances of war and in its immediate aftermath. Despite how badly they were affected, many have purposefully denied their burden of trauma and ignored its psychological consequences. For many, it was only the external push for the required testimonies to legally prosecute the crimes and perpetrators that eventually established forms of communal gathering in which survivors were able to tell their traumatic stories and give witness to the experiences of others. While psychic splitting aimed at preventing the trauma from interfering with postwar recovery and a return to a "normal life," it also helped to nurture what we today recognize as the culture of silence among survivors.

Bar-On (1999) elaborated on the thesis of the "double wall" concerning the children of war survivors who struggle to restore the experiences of their parents' war past, and who are "weaving pieces of historical truth with their fantasies… to create their own imagery of the way the war looked the position their parents had in it and effect it had on people" (Yordanova 2015, 71; see also Auerhahn & Laub 1998). Comparing the study of trauma transmission during times in which information and the evidence of atrocities were left to the strength of the survivors to speak about, and those who had the means to record the testimonies, to today's information and communication technologies, which allow for the restoration of history and the preservation of testimonies, we can see that the transmission of trauma has acquired a very different character. While the descendants of Holocaust survivors were left to the mercy of their parents and grandparents to access any bits of historical truth, today's descendants of survivors might rather want to escape the omnipresence of the evidence.

I claim that today, when Bosnia-Herzegovina has become a global laboratory in which to develop and experiment with memory practices and politics, one must make a conscious decision not to learn about their family histories. The level of knowledge and understanding of these traumatic legacies and how first hand experiences of these traumatic events may endure for future generations is today incomparably more extensive than it was following the Holocaust. Marianne Hirsch writes that it is perhaps only future generations who can fully embrace, witness, and approach the violent events, because they have not lived through them, but rather received them in selected, mediated forms of memory narratives, actions, and symptoms (Hirsch 2012, 12). Generations raised in the aftermath of today's contemporary conflicts have an advantage not only in their temporal (and sometimes spatial) dissociation from these violent pasts. Their advantage in working through trauma lies in their access to information and newly-produced knowledge that were unavailable to both earlier postwar generations and those currently living through conflicts. The children of survivors have access to the embodied, lived experiences of survivors; however, they do not necessarily have the tools – linguistic, discursive, but also representational and symbolic – to work through trauma in ways that are available to succeeding generations and with which with they might actually learn how to avoid repeating the same old mistakes.

If the wars of the 1990s produced any important learning outcome that has the potential to stick with the new generation, it is the need to approach the teaching of history by incorporating those skills of emotional intelligence that are usually taught in other fields of the humanities (philosophy, sociology, psychology). Yet, Bar-On's concept is still extremely interesting, particularly in its understanding of how what is transmitted might be not only genetic, automatic, uncontrolled, and subconscious, but also very purposefully chosen by the younger generation. One such incident happened to me when I stayed at a "war hostel" in Sarajevo in March 2019. I randomly found the place, and despite my generally critical position toward any type of war tourism, I wanted to learn about the place first hand. I booked "a mattress" at a place in Sarajevo that promises you will "experience the war conditions" and where you can hear

> 24/7 original gunfire and bomb sounds from the war (…), there is no electricity (…) for your phones and laptops (…) just a couple of car batteries for the makeshift lights (…) no comfort, you will sleep on the floor on a bomb shelter bed, made of humanitarian blankets used in the war.
>
> (retrieved from the web)

When I booked my "bomb shelter bed," I received an email reply from *Zero One*, whom I eventually met in person when I arrived at the hostel that late night in March 2019. It was off-season, and so the place was empty. I was welcomed at the door by a young man dressed in an army uniform, his head covered with the blue UN helmet. As I am curious about reenactments, I decided to play along. I let him take me inside the house, which did indeed resemble a bomb shelter, only very clean and empty. *Zero One* was talkative and well informed; he gave me a quick, emotionally loaded lecture on the Sarajevo siege, emphasizing that his narrative was important because it came from a survivor. He did not inquire much about my background, so I decided not to interrupt his performance. In fact, I wanted to experience "a service," which he offered to any random tourists coming to stay at this place. I asked questions about his stories rather persistently, and after a couple of hours he escorted me to one of the rooms, where I made my improvisational bed on the floor. As it was early March, it was still winter in Sarajevo, and the room was freezing. The recording of snipers was on repeat the entire night and, as promised in the description online, I had to collect water outside to splash myself a bit after a long trip.

I left the house the next morning for my other work-related errands. Spending the day in a lively, enjoyable city that was full of bars, great food, fashion, and music, I struggled to put my mind back into "war" mode when returning in the evening. On the second night, *Zero One* returned to my "room," we lighted a fire in the old stove, and waited for the water to boil so I could wash myself. Like the previous night, we again engaged in long conversation. It seemed that war as such had deeply consumed him; being born during the siege in 1992, he was fully committed to learning about the siege and to live as a "survivor." This night he was not dressed in uniform, and our conversation grew less official. I shared with him about my work and told him that my visit to this hostel was not for the purpose of "experiencing the war" but rather to experience a reenactment of the war experience. At one point during our conversation I told him that, after leaving his hostel, I would be heading to Foča and to Višegrad and that I would be staying in Vilina Vlas.

In contrast to his encyclopedic knowledge of the Sarajevo siege, he was almost surprised when I told him about the mass rapes and that the Vilina Vlas hotel was most infamously known for being used as a "rape camp" during the war. He had never heard about the hotel and what happened there. He later told me that he had "heard something about rapes" but was not really interested as this was not *his experience* of surviving the war. While he showed interest in the subject by posing some questions, he also became visibly disturbed by me doing this work. As the water boiled, he left so I could wash myself, and when he returned some twenty minutes later I was sure that he had just conducted some online research. We continued talking, but he was now visibly disturbed, trying to convince me that any work related to the legacies of war rapes was hopeless. Especially when done by someone who is not even a survivor, like himself. That night I wrote in my diary:

He kept asking me why I am doing this work and he kept repeating that my work is meaningless as this situation will never change. I asked him why he doesn't live the "normal" life of a twenty-something youngster instead of wearing a UN uniform and embracing the identity of survivor – I admit, I have trouble seeing him as a newborn survivor, though I do believe the war affected him as well – if not while it was going on, certainly in post-war times when he was also more conscious about his surroundings. But the most striking point in our conversation for me was how much trouble he had gone to lead this entire conversation about rape, and even Vilina Vlas. To me this was troubling too – someone who installs bomb recordings for people to "feel" the war has a problem with me going to the actual place where war was happening and is now somehow trying to redefine it.

(Sarajevo, March 2019)[2]

To me, the conversation with *Zero One*, and the entire context of where and how it happened, was important in understanding that trauma transmission is partly a conscious process and a part of memory culture that postwar generations decide to foster. At the same time, I believe that the notion of cultural trauma in this selection process is not enough, because young people would not necessarily feel the past when experiencing the same or similar traumatic symptoms as their parents. While the rapes seemed incomprehensible to this young man, he had built his entire *personal* (survivor) and *professional* (war tourism service provider) identity around pieces that he had collected from his parents and from other *chosen* sources. While he did not search for sources regarding the Vilina Vlas case, he possessed more knowledge about the siege of Sarajevo than his parents, who had consciously lived and experienced it. As I had a chance to briefly converse with his parents, it was very obvious that he is far more resourceful than they were. In accordance with Bar-On's double wall concept, *Zero One* has successfully emptied the spaces of his parents' shared memories – but not merely with all the information he could find and collect. The gaps were filled with selected information – the information that helped him build the identity that serves his personal and professional purposes.

Another example happened during my 2018 stay in Srebrenica, where I accompanied a group of youngsters as they visited an abandoned factory in Potočari on their mission to find remains of the massacre. While walking there, one of the young men mentioned to me that "some people are talking about the 'blood room', a room where one can supposedly see a bloody handprint on the wall 'from someone who was executed'" (from fieldnotes, 2018). This information is confusing because the former car battery factory, which is today partly reconstructed as a memorial center and gallery and partly abandoned, did not serve as a place of execution. It was – at least in theory – a safe area, a base for Dutch UN peacekeepers that became a refuge for local people after the fall of Srebrenica. However, I did not intervene as I wanted to learn what information and knowledge the students possessed and, more importantly, why they were so keen to find signs of torture and violent atrocity. As it transpired, they were on a mission to find famous graffiti left by Dutch soldiers, but they were also very eager to find any human remains and were disappointed that no such remains existed.

While passing the largest hall, I spotted "bones" on the floor that were the remains of the *One Million Bones* project installed in Potočari in 2015.[3] The three youngsters were very excited about the discovery, taking photos and posting them on social media. They shared their discoveries with others when we returned to the camp. Observing and reflecting on the experiences of those three young people, I felt that I was not entitled to judge or condemn their approach to the Srebrenica issue. As far as possible, I tried to remain a neutral observer, merely asking questions during and after the visit and in later informal conversations. This served as my springboard for discussing and understanding aspects of the violent past.

However, it is challenging to deny their overall emotional fascination with the site, and especially with learning more about mass murder, bones, bloody remains, and torture. It is even more challenging to present, analyze, and discuss this – here, in the present paper – without it seeming that I am accusing these young people of some type of "war porn." When talking about this experience with their fellows in the camp, the excitement was evident in their body language, attitudes, and narratives. In their study, Firangiz Israfilova and Catherny Khoo-Lattimore found similar responses from the analysis of children visiting the Guba Genocide Memorial Complex in Azerbaijan; while most felt sad, there were some who were fascinated and enjoyed the visit (2018, 8). What led those three young people into the halls of the factory was a search for something they could identify with, an experience embodied in fellow human bodies – the pain and suffering of fellow human beings and the experience of survival. Perhaps they also felt the thrill of connecting with the past through finding concrete remains. Finding a bloody handprint on the wall is finding *real* evidence that *real* people were here – that these people, in fact, are not only numbers and a long list of names. And finding blood means those people were there not long ago. One of them told me that what interests them are the "stories":

> We have never heard this in school. They told us the facts. I know everything about who was fighting, who was killed, when this happened, but being here in Srebrenica, for me, means much more. Suddenly it feels so real. I am very excited. I could return to this factory over and over again.
>
> (from a conversation, July 2018)

They returned four more times. On those visits, they were neither shocked nor intimidated; rather, they were entertained, as they would be at an amusement park, not knowing exactly what awaited them except the adrenaline and the thrill – the excitement. There is no such excitement in learning about the rapes and how to memorialize the traumatic history of the survivors, or in learning from young people that their parents did not want to share anything at home. From my own experience of bringing this topic to the table, there is almost always the same strange silence among youth when conversation turns to rape and the survivors. I am not trying to say that young people were always open about or constructive toward learning about the past. Also, my own practice is very limited in its scope as to how many peace education programs are organized annually in the entire country. Yet, in considering the evidence available to me, rape has never been brought into the discussion. I have met and conversed with youth who knew about their parents and their war stories, but there was never anything related to sexual violence. Moreover, when witnessing the excitement of these youth as they discovered the remains of Srebrenica, I began to think, *How can I apply this experience to similar places that were known for rapes?* Would "rape remains" generate the same excitement? Was the fact that this youth had no family in Srebrenica or in the region during the war a safeguard against feeling too much pain or emotional attachment while learning about the violent past?

Srebrenica has gained a special place in Bosnian and international memory culture, and its politics have been disputed on several levels and approached through different narratives (Simić 2009; Halilovich 2015; Jacobs 2016). However, prioritized interest and the simultaneous and long-term neglect of other, less notorious war contexts (or refusal to acknowledge genocidal acts elsewhere in Bosnia-Herzegovina) have transformed Srebrenica into a metaphysical, if not surreal, place. The annual commemoration becomes a form of reenactment, with the mothers – dressed in traditional clothing, with props of green coffins and a huge audience witnessing their sorrow, grief, and mourning – as protagonists. Young people share in the mourning, but a visit to the memorial site also generates excitement. Like Auschwitz, Srebrenica now risks becoming a "Disneyland of Misery."[4] The mass execution in Srebrenica or, similarly, the siege of Sarajevo, gives the impression that the scale of these events and the memory, the remains, the legacy, can be seized and, in a way, controlled.

On the other hand, mass rapes were happening all over; anyone could be affected, the estimated number of 20,000–50,000 victims is big. While one can visit Srebrenica or the war hostel in Sarajevo and leaves one's emotions and the experience there, outside of the home, the legacy of war rapes might be right there in the very center of everyone's homes. While the youth that I spoke with were usually open to discussing the war and the ways in which the war was spoken about at home, I always had trouble trying to discuss the rapes. I noted that this difference was established in general war-related communication, not only during my ethnographic work, but also whenever I presented my work at professional events where other experts dealt with different aspects of memory culture and the traumatic legacies of war. The topic of war rapes, particularly in relation to the mothers, those mothers who live and mother today, was almost always met with a strange silence.

Dan Bar-On (2006) recognizes how dissociation in the form of silence can be functional and helpful in the direct aftermath of war also to prevent transmission of traumas; however, in later stages, he claims that "the same silencing becomes dysfunctional, especially when it leads to intergenerational transmission of the effects of physical or moral trauma" (Bar-On 2006, 37). It is then that storytelling becomes a crucial practice for processing collective traumas, healing, and social reintegration (of both the story and the survivor). Most parents strive, as do the survivors, to transmit to their offspring only those parts of the culture that they have approved, which can sometimes manifest in a "mirror image" (Bertaux & Thompson 2005, 2). But again, as the transmission is a two-way process – from parents to children and vice versa – and at the same time an individual and collective process, family – particularly mothers – might have a certain level of control as to what may be handed down, but not absolute control. More than unconscious transmissions – which are hard to control, stop, or prevent – one might consider the preoccupation and expectation of the survivors that the descendants should show the interest and actively participate in commemoration and remembrance practices initiated, organized and led by survivors. While for the survivors, their memory culture is perhaps central to their postwar lives and social reintegration, imposing these same activities to the youth might actually result in negative responses of youth. Overtime, the irritation that initially comes from the pressure of their parents *to remember* and *not to forget* the violent past, transforms to the ideologies of revenge, inter-group hatred, and rejecting constructive and critical learning of anything related to the violent past, hence, *the past of their parents*. As I will try to show in the last section of the book, if listening to youth and giving them space to create their own "memory," the future might seem much brighter than the one offered by disappointed, frustrated, and mostly trauma-bound survivors.

War-rape legacies in (peace) education

Since the mid-1990s, Bosnia-Herzegovina has been one of the most donor-dense countries in Eastern Europe, and the number of peace building and reconciliation activities that have been conducted both by international stakeholders and local grass-roots organizations is vast (Orford 2003; Parent 2016). So are the scholarly resources that reflected on the projects on the ground, but also projected new opportunities would help communities to reunite despite the state's continuous efforts on all levels – discursive, symbolic, physical – to keep them divided. International efforts for peace building particularly received a great deal of criticism, and despite the efforts by different agents to diminish the power imbalance between the international interventions and local grass-roots activism, top-down externally delegated norms and approaches to peace building and reconciliation have importantly shaped today's manner of dealing with the traumatic legacies in even the postwar generations (Paris 2004; Richmond 2004; Zanotti 2006):

> In Bosnia and Herzegovina, outsiders do more than participate in shaping the political agenda /.../ In BiH outsiders actually *set* that agenda, *impose* it, and *punish with sanctions* those who refuse to implement it.
>
> (Knaus and Martin 2003, 61)

In *Muscular Interventionism*, Maria O'Reilly writes about international peace building and reconciliation interventions in a gendered and orientalist manner, where the international community, as "heroic, altruistic, white males," is on a mission to "protect the vulnerable, inferior, feminized 'other'" (O'Reilly 2012, 545). According to her, peace projects (re)produce a gendered, classed, and Balkanized (racialized) order in which "manliness" and "Western-ness" are both signifiers and sources of privilege, superiority, and domination. Other writers, mainly feminists, have criticized the leading approaches to peace building as being limited to a male point of view, as the end of the war does not necessarily mean the end of other types of violence in society (Porter 2007, 28–29). For a lot of survivors, official peace agreements did end the military intervention but the war-related violence continued at their home – either in the form of social repercussions such as stigma and ostracism or as male violence coming from traumatized spouses. However, for many survivors, domestic violence was a return "back to normal" as they were trained through the formal school system and at home to normalize certain forms of violence. The understanding of peace is, therefore, often subject to male-defined norms and values (see, e.g., Brock-Utne 1985, 33).

While most of the criticisms of peace building and reconciliation in Bosnia-Herzegovina have focused on the ideologies that are being welcomed mostly due to the generous financial support, I would also emphasize that many grass-roots organizations and informal groups of individuals are not only passively accepting the dictated order from donors. On the contrary, many have learned very well how to create their own space beyond the donors' influence and how to assert their agendas independently from their donors' total control. From my own peace education practice, I believe that while critical reflection on international intervention through some kind of (post, neo)colonial lens keeps theoreticians and practitioners alert and questioning "imported" practices, the processes of peace building and reconciliation are live mechanisms that sooner or later adjust to the needs of the local environments. They take on the local character that then distinguishes them from previous versions and those "developed in the West" or adopted in other cultural and political contexts.

Reconciliation processes generally consist of legal frameworks of retributive (perpetrator- and punishment-centered) and restorative (victim- and reparation-centered) justice and operates between internationally agreed upon solutions toward the end, where the legacies of the conflict and local needs and challenges are related to traumas at individual, collective, and national levels (see Francis 2002; Eastmond 2010; Nordquist 2017). National reconciliation is achieved when the social and political situations stabilize enough to prevent reverting to the old patterns of conflict or revenge fantasy. Individual reconciliation is the ability of those who participated, witnessed, and/or survived the war and those who were born into the war torn society in the aftermath of the conflict to conduct their lives similarly to the way they did before the conflict, without hate, fear, or avoidance (Mobekk 2005, 263). In the frame of peace building, reconciliation relates to trauma healing, teaching ways of dealing with the past, rebuilding interethnic and inter-religious communication and cooperation, and promoting peaceful coexistence. Ideally, the early stages of rebuilding communities and assessing the scope of crimes and casualties should be followed by attempts at forgiveness, community work, and economic and political development (Nordquist 2006; Schaap 2008; Brown et al. 2010;).

Empirically, this calls for the communities that are interested in expressing and exercising their will to actively participate in crossing the comfort zones of the divided places, to face the pain of the other, and to recreate social values, practices, and future aspirations that will respond to the needs of all. Reconciliation leads to sustainable inter-group relationships only if the involved parties acquaint themselves with acknowledging each other's interpretation of the traumatic events, which also means that they learn how to tackle controversies and where perpetrators should take a lead in addressing the wrongdoings committed during the conflict (Auerbach 2009; Jansen 2013).

While the process of reconciliation is always happening on several levels simultaneously, in the scope of the ethnographic research here, I mainly reflect on what is known as "thick" reconciliation, which refers to the emotional components of local, bottom-up practices of trauma healing with a victim-centered approach (Eastmond 2010; Hoogenbom & Vieille 2010; Bloomfield 2016). International interventions in the aftermath of a conflict obviously impact the understanding and approaches to healing, restorative justice, democratization, and institutional development in retributive justice and punishment of the perpetrators. Yet I believe that those practices always get localized and adopted within a specific sociocultural environment of the groups dealing with it and their capacities, skills, and knowledge. While thick reconciliation includes grass-roots actors, it primarily refers to organized activism, with individuals and collectives who are knowledgeable and resourceful enough to recruit, motivate, and mobilize local populations in their work. In the previous chapters, I have approached the understanding of building "peace from below," which pays careful attention to the local context and views local culture and knowledge as resources (Lederach 1997) in the context of trauma healing and mothering with trauma among the survivors of war-related sexual violence, as (first) providers of peace education. If peace education is a commitment to end any type of violence and to quest for ending inequalities, including sexism, is it therefore a responsibility of mothers–survivors, those who have firsthand experience of the radical violent manifestations of the power of sexism, to resist to raise their offspring in the patriarchal mode. Are the mothers who survived the atrocities to be blamed for not learning anything from the past if they fear the rape of their daughters and transfer this fear? One of the mothers would respond in this way:

> My fear is raising him /her son/ in hatred because I feel responsible. I taught him to walk, to talk, and how to behave during a meal. What would make me think that I am not teaching him also love and hate? I know he is his own human, but at the end, we mothers are the first to tell our kids about the world.
>
> (L, September 2018, North Bosnia)

The other adds to the same conversation:

> I am not responsible for what happened to me. I am not responsible for my husband beating me. He is a pig. But for my /names omitted/, it is only me who can teach them what is good and what is bad. And I will not raise them in bad. I am not even telling them anything bad about their father, even though he is a pig. He will get his own punishment, a good God sees everything.
>
> (R, September 2018, North Bosnia)

Despite the general agreement among theoreticians, practitioners, and local communities about the necessity for forgiving, reconciling, and moving on in order to guarantee a stable and secure future, empirical implementations of those plans are much more challenging. This is most simply reflected in the gap between donors' expectations and project realization in the field, where the impact and tangible results may not be easily measured or seen within the time frame and funding limits of a project over a couple of years. Donors are usually not integrated in the everyday life and dynamics of the local organizations, which sometimes results in a paternalistic, postcolonial nature to an imbalanced power relationship. For example, the very case of war-related sexual violence, its legacy, and current efforts to position it within the existing peace education programs or perhaps event critical history curricula shows a time span of its dynamics in the field of sociopolitical discourse (from silence and stigma to brave and strong heroines–survivors) and collective memory (from victims to survivors).

While the early narratives on powerless and silent victims have proved harmful, the new perspectives on the topic might help us to emphasize the critical understanding of the phenomena of collective victimhood and victimization as such. The immense contribution in terms of epistemological knowledge in the field can help us extract pedagogical particles to be integrated in teaching. In retrospect, the development of this knowledge also emphasizes the remaining obstacles and perhaps threats for the survivors and their families that may be presented by education in war-rape legacies. In addition to the criticism related to the unequal power relationship and domination built mostly on financial support, the past scholarship has also been critical of the obvious rivalry and competition that limited funding causes among local stakeholders (see, e.g., Bieber 2002; Parent 2016; Bajramović 2018).

From my experience as well, this presents perhaps the biggest obstacle to reconciling, forgiving, and peace building. At the same time, I understand there are multifaceted obstacles to such cooperation that do not necessarily originate in an inability to have a multi-perspectivity and understanding of the other side of the story. The war was waged in very different formats, for instance, and have affected communities in different ways – so different that, sometimes, survivors would even talk about several simultaneous wars that were waged in different areas of the country. Very often, I have encountered situations where I was more informed about the scope of the violence in other areas than survivors themselves. Specifically, an inability to collaborate is within the efforts of many social groups and organizations trying to find the "truth" of the events in their own context. Between the denial and the slow justice processes on national level, this therefore demands full-time engagement. In addition, "the other side" is not necessarily defined only by the ethno-religious identity of those who today are perceived as "former perpetrators." The other side might be simply groups of survivors who have differently defined goals in restorative and retributive justice. Elsewhere in this book, I gave the example of mothers from Srebrenica and mothers who are war-rape survivors that define their missions in very different terms and rarely see the need to collaborate or unite their efforts against the oppressive and denying system. Defining a nationwide reconciliation that could respond to the needs of all these very differently wounded communities is therefore a rather ambitious goal.

I have worked for several years as a youth worker in a field where I could define peace education: antidiscrimination and social justice education, prevention of violence, antiracism, and hate speech prevention. Since 2011, I have focused more on research related to the social recovery of war-rape survivors and started to work in formal education at university; however, I remain active in informal education, trying to connect the legacies of war-related rapes and sexual violence in so-called peace times. Before starting field research for this project in 2017, I had been following the social media and home pages of various nongovernmental organizations that work in the field of youth work and peace education, and lately, also what is now recognized as a critical history education. After getting myself familiar with the work that includes young generations who are very different from older survivors that were participating in my previous research, I believed that working with youth would be more motivating in terms of a brighter, trauma-free future and would thus affect me less, particularly in terms of secondary trauma. On the contrast to the focus of the survivors that mainly look back, most of the peace education activities for youth are focused on the future. I was particularly looking for possibilities to unite these two perspectives of past and future in a new pedagogical stream.

When I introduced the project and my ideas to the survivors and discussed the possibilities to invite them to collaborate in peace education programs, they responded in a very positive and enthusiastic way. This was, indeed, very different from my past experiences with them, where I was focused mostly on their own (i.e., survivors as isolated individuals) recovery process, the narratives, and their (re)integration back into their local communities. Before, they never really showed much interest, or perhaps better said, they never showed any belief or hope that yet another project would change their destiny and their (political) efforts for better in any way. They had invested a lot of energy in the previous years to break down the stigma and to affect positive social change in this matter, but their efforts were mostly met with ignorance from society or a passive and slow response from the state institutions in charge. The motivation coming from survivors made me reflect on the dispersed nature of the reconciliatory work mentioned above beyond what most critics would note, namely competition and conflicting agendas that are based mostly on different and contradictory interpretations of the past (see Kappler 2013). For women survivors, working with youth was a fresh and new idea, without previously engaging in it, particularly because their own interests and political agendas were primarily attached to the survivors' related rights, status, and compensation. The outcomes and benefits that they expect from their work toward reconciliation are essentially different from, for instance, veterans, former medical or police staff, descendants of missing individuals, and so on. And last but not least, from the aspirations that today's youth might have when looking into the future, *their* future. After a visit to one of the associations I have been in contact with since 2013, I wrote the following in my diary:

> In the morning, I was all bitter, and I was ready for them to again be tired of new proposals and new engagement. That they will perhaps enjoy this visit

and conversation we will have, but they will, of course, not really see how my idea of working with youth could enhance their social status or bring any changes in terms of dealing with the social aspects of their traumas. They completely surprised me: they agreed on the importance of working with youth, and they were immediately ready to travel to other parts of the country and have a workshop with youth. That really motivated me, also in the very thought of why I hadn't thought of such intergenerational work between survivors and post-war youth before. Why are the survivors following their own agendas within their associations, and teachers and other educators are addressing the survivors' legacy through second-hand views?

(Central Bosnia, March 2018)

Many individuals and social groups are therefore engaged in remembrance practices and reconciliation processes, but they never meet across the interethnic/inter-religious, and/or intergenerational lines. For survivors, remembrance is often a pragmatic effort to achieve justice and, more importantly, against denying the crimes (e.g., Manegrem Selimovic 2013; McGrattan & Hopkins 2016). This is an important component of *their* wider agenda; however, it does not necessarily also align with the agenda of their descendants or the postwar generation in general. One can assume that because (grand)parents share their war stories in families, the youth will be attached to this history to the same extent. Survivors assume that new generations that have never experienced war can simply work on empathic connections and thus develop the ability to commemorate "war" as the survivors want it to be remembered. Mother–survivors told me that they want their offspring and other postwar youth to remember and know their history, the history of their family and not the history of the war from the books.

But are the memories created and nurtured by survivors primarily important for survivors, or can these same memories in fact be meaningful for the postwar youth (either descendants or not)? While survivors (might) play an important role in creating and guarding the grand narratives of memory, how do young people contribute to this process? Finally, do young people really need (or want) to remember? What would their motivation for remembrance be? Is remembering so as not to repeat past atrocities really the goal of such intergenerational transmission of memory, or is this the goal of those who survived or witnessed the war? And last but not least, what is there to remember and learn from the sexual violence used as a weapon of war? Sometimes, as I could also hear during my brief teaching experiences in 2018 and 2019, the youth simply do not care. Perhaps they would if they felt that they could actively co-create the memory and with their own interpretation that is positively received by the survivors, too. During one of the workshops with teenagers between 15 and 17 years of age in July 2018, we were discussing a commemoration in Srebrenica, and one of the students commented that he had noticed posts on Facebook but had scrolled through because he "knew this already." He added that he "didn't learn anything new." I asked other students in the group whether it was important to have news about Srebrenica's annual commemoration in the newspaper every year, and one student responded

> It is an important day, and of course newspapers will report on it. From these newspapers, I didn't learn anything new because I have seen pictures from Srebrenica before. I still think it is important to remind us, and I also think that many people do not know about this, because it is very far from us and it also happened a very long time ago.
>
> (K, July 2018, Mostar)

In order to avoid violating the code of "appropriating" the remembrance practices created by survivors, youth would sometimes feel it was safer to adhere to what was expected of them, without any critical appraisal or reflection. However, every generation (mis)uses the collective memory in its own way, despite how survivors would like the impact to be and to dictate the *appropriate, desired memory consumption*.

After the positive response from the survivors and their motivation to be included in peace education with youth, we planned to deliver a pilot workshop with youth in a school in a town different from their hometown (for the survivors to feel safer). The workshop, that I mentioned briefly elsewhere in the book, was finally organized in November 2018 and was attended by fifteen youths and two survivors. We allocated most of the time for the survivors to speak in smaller groups, to share their testimonies and answer questions from the youths, but also introducing the youth to the adjusted versions of "pyramid of hate," where they could reflect on different layers and forms of (sexual violence), particularly those that are being kept invisible and are being normalized (like sexist jokes, mansplaining, and catcalling, for instance). In this part of the workshop, the youth were also invited to reflect in the vein of Stanton's eight stages of genocide (1996), which would reveal war-related rapes as a nonlinear and complex multistage process rather than an isolated war crime. In addition, the idea of defining the "preceding stages" of the war rapes, such as normalized marital rape or nonconsensual relationships, was to aid understanding of the existence of a rape culture through historical contexts and in times of peace.[5]

At the end of the workshop, we gathered back in the plenary, where the youth were asked to share their impressions and the "learning experiences from the past," combining it with the triangle model of adjusted "pyramid of hate" to address what they could take with them, but also to reflect on today's social issues related to sexual and gender-based violence. For all of the students, encountering a survivor of war rape and being able to hear her story firsthand was a powerful experience. They posed a lot of questions, most of which related to the survivors' statuses today and how they dealt with perpetrators who were still free. In the final feedback, the participating youth did not provide any concrete ideas for how to use these historical experiences to prevent future cycles of violence, which I believe was due more to lack of time and the overwhelming experience that this encounter was for them than to a lack of feedback. They agreed that such encounters are important and that they should happen more often. The same sentiments also came from the school staff present at the workshop.

When I was driving the two survivors back to their home, which was a more than four hour ride in the car, I had a great chance to listen to their impressions and their feedback. For them, the entire experience was unique and very fulfilling in terms of positive self-esteem. One of them was explaining that she is often frustrated talking to general audiences or journalists because she feels no one is listening. Conversely, when she was sitting among the curious young people who were so active with questions, she felt that perhaps they are the audience she should speak to more often. Both also mentioned that they were surprised how much respect they felt coming from the youth, their acknowledgment, and the way they received the stories, particularly because they had really feared that the youngsters were too young for such types of testimonies. After four hours, I dropped them off, tired but in a very positive mood, and in the following days, I received an email from the leader of the association that was full of positive feedback and proposed repeating this workshop and also engaging other members of the organization.

The positive and curious response from the youth during the workshop and the survivors' positive feedback might indicate the prospects and importance of intergenerational work between survivors and postwar youth, and that could lead to some completely new directions in peace and reconciliation work on both sides. Both the survivors and the youth were invited into a space of mutual exchange where the outcomes and goals of the workshop were not definitely set; the youth could ask questions but also comment. With the help of the pyramid of hate model, they were invited to position the testimonies in the context of sexual violence perpetuated today and explore different (invisible) formats that in the end would allow the systematic use of rapes in the conflict, and moreover, that allows the effective employment of long-term social repercussions such as stigma and ostracism. The positive mutual exchange and the acknowledgment of different departure points between survivors and postwar youths also happened during a visit to Foča that I describe elsewhere in this book.

The successfully implemented pilot workshops were a good reference point from which I could approach other youth and peace workers in my efforts to establish future collaborations. However, I have encountered a rather unexpected silence and nonresponsiveness from most of the potential partners I wanted to reach out to. First, I approached an organization that is one of the most visible and active youth organizations and deals mostly with sexuality and gender-related topics with a great emphasis on the prevention of sexual violence. They invited me for a visit, where we briefly discussed their current programs, and I got acquainted with their rich and regular publications from the field. Without question, their contribution to the field of sex education is important and valuable, but it does not engage with the testimonies or the legacy of mass rapes during the conflict in general. There is no special focus in their agenda for drawing correlations between the sexual scripts in times of war and peace. They are strongly connected to feminist groups in the broader Western Balkans region, and have a connection to those feminist activists that were particularly prominent in the 1990s as well as in the women's antiwar demonstrations in Belgrade.

I mentioned the pilot workshops and the idea of implementing such programs in more systematic way. I also shared my ideas on the importance of intergenerational work and the possibilities of engaging mother–survivors in peace education and sexual violence prevention programs. However, they never provided me with any reaction or clear response to my ideas. As I kept insisting with my questions, the representative told me that "survivors have their own organizations where they deal with their issues" (field notes 2019) and she directed me to the most well recognized, the *Association* of Women *Victims* of *War*. I tried to elaborate further that my interest is not in the agenda of survivors' organizations, but rather in potential collaborations that would be based on the intergenerational transmission of knowledge, experiences, and the mutual exchange of understanding of sexuality, gender, and violence in peace and war, but I still got no interest from them.

Despite this initial failure, I remain determined to get in contact with other organizations, so I first wrote to the organization that annually hosts a peace education summer camp, first only inquiring about their programs and how much the topic of sexual violence is included in their working agenda. When they responded that they did not have any existing program but believe it is an important topic to address, I offered to join as a volunteer to be able to observe by participation, and the program coordinator was enthusiastic about this collaboration. However, soon afterward, he informed me – without any detailed explanation – that it was no longer possible and that, unfortunately, the workshops we had planned would not be possible to deliver. Although respecting this sudden decision, I still followed their program through their social media and learned that they indeed had a workshop on sexual violence and nationalism, led by a fellow foreign researcher. I have tried to get in contact with this researcher to learn how they addressed the topic and also the response from the participants or perhaps any survivors who were involved in the session. Unfortunately, I have never received a response.

My emails and calls remained unanswered with two other organizations, one of which collaborated with UNFPA on the drama projects that I will discuss in the next section. From what I was able to obtain without their input, I learned that they have started to incorporate the topic of sexual violence and its related stigma in their programs; however, I was not able to obtain any data or second-hand evidence regarding what aspects and how they approached the teaching. The one positive response that I got was from the director of one the biggest youth work and informal education networks that unites 178 local organizations and twenty-one schools. In the conversation, he welcomed the idea of working together with the survivors of sexual violence and also assured me that he was not familiar with any other such projects despite being active in peace education since the early years after the war. With further research into some of his references, I could only draw vague conclusions that the topic of sexual violence is getting more recognition also in youth work. Still, to the best of my knowledge, there are not many with direct cooperation between survivors and postwar youths.

The failure to get responses from most organizations left me quite frustrated, especially after the positive experience of the pilot workshop with survivors. In addition, this leaves me with very little ethnographic evidence beyond my own experience for building up the existing curricula in peace education and prevention of sexual violence that would draw particularly on intergenerational work between mother–survivors and postwar youths. Why so much insistence on such a collaboration? I believe my most important motivation lies in adopting the mothers' most expressed position that past experiences, including trauma, might indeed be transmitted and have a negative impact on their offspring if not resolved or purposefully addressed. Therefore, in our efforts as teachers to break the cycles of violence, we need to start approaching the processes of trauma transmission in families through more systematic pedagogical approaches, meaning not leaving the trauma transmission to its unconscious nature or remaining unspoken, not having a language and perception of it as a random, uncontrolled process within socialization, where each individual works toward its prevention (or not) to the best of their ability.

I believe that acknowledging the transmission and its manifestations in the behavioral and relational patterns of everyday life through the conscious process of engaged learning would help us as teachers to develop preventive mechanisms together with the survivors (bearing the firsthand experience of trauma) and the postwar generations (witnessing and coping with the legacies). During my work, I have met a number of individuals – survivors, practitioners, fellow researchers, and youth – who all agreed to some extent that learning from the past is important for preventing similar circumstances in the future. Yet, no one was really clear on what *we can actually learn* from the mass use of rape and sexual violence during the conflict in the 1990s. Stressing the importance of intergenerational learning, not only within families but also in the framework of formal educational programs assumes that generations in the aftermath of war, the generations born to survivors, *must remember* and must carry on the legacy and memory of survivors even after all of them vanish, mostly with the argument of not forgetting *them* and *their* pain.

But what if forgetting and letting the memory of the survivors is exactly what one needs to do to build their own social order and power relationships? One particularly consistent response from the youth in my 2018 workshop concerned the need to stop talking about the past, bringing it up repeatedly instead of looking forward. One of the students told me:

I am really tired of these war stories. I want to live my life and just move on. Sometimes, I feel I can't think who I am because I need to listen what happened before me. Of course, I want to know what happened, but I am also tired because it never stops. I don't think this is my history, and therefore, I would be happy to be spared listening to it over and over again.

(L16, South Bosnia 2018)

Nonetheless, teachers and students in an unstable postconflict environment struggle to openly discuss the violent past – even in very general terms of history, not specifically with regard to sexual violence used in conflict. In one of the workshops, I asked underage participants for their parents' permission to use the outcomes produced during the workshop in my research materials. While obtaining consent is typically performed as part of a procedure in any research with human participants, it is a rather unusual practice in the classroom while also teaching. All but one set of parents gave their signed consent. Another student came to me with his signed consent form and told me that although his parents had signed the form, "They do not want me to talk much about what happened during the war, and they want me to leave the class if we talk about it too much" (P14, Southeast Bosnia 2018). This same student did not participate in any of the activities that were related to the recent war. He remained in the room, but left his papers blank. After the class, I invited him to talk to me and share how he felt. He said,

> I feel OK. I like this class. I just have no idea of what to draw or write when you ask me. I don't feel bad or like I don't want to write or join in. I just have no ideas.
>
> (P14, Southeast Bosnia 2018)

To run this workshop, I responded to the call for volunteer teaching staff for the Mostar Summer Youth Programme (MSYP) with the intention of taking the continuation of violence in a historical perspective as my subject. The main coordinator shared my ideas with other staff at the school, and they all expressed hesitancy about the subject and stressed the need for a cautious approach when teaching about the recent violent history of Mostar. These concerns have been previously debated by educators who found themselves in a postconflict context not specifically focused on or related to peace building education, particularly history and language teachers in state schools who struggle to remain just and critical in coping with emotionally demanding content (see Pavlowitch 2004; Murphy & Gallagher 2009; McCully 2012). Cole and Barsalou (2006), for instance, write how in similar situations, most educators responded with collective amnesia as a way of preventing destabilization of fragile dynamics in the classroom. As the school staff generally agreed that in long run, amnesia is not a constructive approach to dealing with the past, we negotiated to adjust the language policies, beginning by replacing the term *collective violence* with *social oppression*. The latter term can also relate to everyday practices such as prejudice, sexual harassment, and bullying and is supposedly less provocative in this context than collective violence. This would allow the students to respond to the topics that they felt comfortable with and avoid causing distress to their families. Careful handling with potentially triggering trauma among students has been emphasized in trainings of teachers in postconflict environments. Educational programs and pedagogic methods should be sensitive to sources of dispute and ensure a no-harm policy to maintain peace and stability (Smith 2011, 4).

For further recommendations on designing a curriculum related to a violent past, I followed the conceptual framework and model of impact of history education on social identity developed by Karina Korostelina (2013). To expand her thesis on ingroup identity and justification of power structures and social hierarchies (2013, 19–45), I used the concepts of intersectionality and multiple identities, which elucidate how ideological and propagandist strategies employ social exclusion, incorporate discrimination, and sometimes eliminate entire groups. In her study *History Education in Post-Conflict Societies*, Sirkka Ahonen (2014) provides a comparative account of three violent historical events in the three different geographic and political cases of Finland, Bosnia-Herzegovina, and South Africa. While she acknowledged the risks of comparing historically different societies (2014, 83), she also points out the importance of inclusivity, as "history lessons need to incorporate idiosyncratic histories of many groups" (Ahonen 2014, 76). The importance of recognizing past societies in different parts of the world to be able to critically understand and position a view of the history of your own community has been emphasized in studies of historical empathy (see, e.g., Davis, Yeager, & Foster 2001).

Those scholars insist that in order to come to terms with the past and break the cycles of violence, students need to learn to recognize similar patterns and shared values in other (past) societies, to contextualize events in time and place, and to comprehend that multiple perspectives are not to always be contested but also simultaneously acknowledged (D'Adamo & Fallace 2011). The general struggle to freely speak their minds reflects the struggle with breaking the silence that powerfully perpetuates the public narrative of the entire Bosnian society when it comes to the war. Silence in (history) education is one of the most persistent coping mechanisms not only among survivors but generally in postwar contexts, hence breaking the silence is at the core of social action and research of many educators, activists, and individual agents (Igreja 2008; Vinitzky-Seroussi 2010; Winter 2010). However, I would not simplify the occurrence of silence only on the theme but also that the majority of students were exposed to very common postcommunist institutional teaching that incorporated lectures and the Freirean model of banking education, which minimizes students' creative powers and capacity for independent and critical thinking (for more about this, see Freire 1970, 72–74).

At this point, I want to mention that this type of lecturing does not facilitate the transfer of knowledge to different contexts. It does not encourage students to understand, emotionally and cognitively, the many aspects of individual and collective action before, during, and after the particular historical event, historical legacy, and the power of transferred historical memory. By not only their verbal responses but also their emotional reactions and body language during the activities, it was clear that the format of interactive workshops where they were invited to share opinions demanded a different way of engaging. In a closing activity at this same workshop, I asked the participants to write a letter to people "on the other side of the conflict." I did not ask them to write a letter of forgiveness; instead, I asked them to write down what would they like to know from the others, what issues they were curious to explore, and what puzzling questions they would like to address. There were two unexpected outcomes: despite no directions being given, seven (the majority) of the letters concerned the need to forgive and work together for a peaceful future. All of the letters were written in English. In answer to my question about language choice, one of the students told me, "I did not want to be recognized and judged. I wanted to write freely about my thoughts, without thinking about being judged for who I am" (M16, Southeast Bosnia 2018).

In further conversation, more of the participants expressed the burden of the past and how they would like to focus on the problems of their times, especially mass emigration, corruption, and unemployment, instead of focusing on not forgetting their parents' past (field work notes 2018). They claimed that they are often expected to respond to the commemorative needs of those who survived the atrocities with very particular "right," proper, and socially desirable commemorative practices. Public spaces, like the media, always have target audiences and are often subject to market needs, having to provide customers with what they want. Hence, the images and narratives found in the media are designed to satisfy the audience rather than problematize issues and/or keep stories simple. The reality, on the other hand, changes daily as new trials are held, new mass graves are discovered, and new evidence is provided. As generations pass away, consumers of the memory eventually change, and the descendants of survivors become the active readers. But the question is whether anyone wants them to be read as they would like stories to be read.

Several scholars have provided important evidence relating to the teaching of history and war studies in postconflict settings (Pašalić-Kreso 2008; Berkerman & Zembylas 2011; Ahonen 2012). The official history teaching material in Bosnia-Herzegovina, for instance, has been under critical scrutiny since the early stages of the Dayton peace agreement. The use of three different ethnically oriented textbooks has been problematized and has encouraged the establishment of an inclusive textbook that aims to "remove offensive material from textbooks" and introduce modifications to meet "modern European standards" (Karge & Batarilo 2008, 10). With little progress being made, fundamental changes are still needed in terms of curricular harmonization and teacher training for the delivery of content that promotes sociopolitical unity in a diverse Bosnian society. While regulatory regimes, bureaucratic practices, and political will are slow to adopt multiperspectivity in history education, grass-roots organizations are doing important work in engaging different layers of society with different approaches and methods. However, collaboration between institutional and informal education is rather poor (beyond just the Bosnian and postconflict contexts). In contrast to formal history teaching, the noninstitutional programs pay more attention to the study of collective memory and emotional aspects in their approach to violent pasts.[6]

When it comes to teaching about sexual violence, I wonder if it is more important to draw correlations with other cases in history, for instance with Rwanda and now with Yazidi women, or is it more important to draw correlations with the so-called normalized sexual violence in everyday life and how to connect it to the radical uses in the conflict. While mentioning other geographically and historically comparable cases, I see more importance in contextualizing these events in the situation today. Another factor that I noted is the importance of teaching history by incorporating historical events in the broader context of the humanities and social sciences rather than teaching them separately and decontextualizing them. My own background in social and political science is beneficial for explaining historical events from the perspective of social phenomena. Among other examples, I might use the systemic use of rape and sexual violence in the war to reflect on wider gender-based and sexual oppression, both in the past and today, in peace and in conflict. We still fail miserably to understand the phenomena of Auschwitz and Srebrenica as social and political phenomena rather than merely historical ones, and this is exactly where I see the importance of creating diverse collective memories, ethnically and generationally.

Since history is often burdensome for survivors, they should be given the opportunity to first focus fully on their own recovery, leaving the postwar generation in charge of creating the future. However, I do not believe that the postwar generations can create an alternate future if they are continuously exposed to pressure to remember the past and engage in remembrance practices of older generations with other agendas. While for the survivors, achieving justice is one of the most important incentives for insisting on certain memorial narratives, for young people, it is important to understand not only who the victims and perpetrators were or how many and which people were killed, but how individual human beings anywhere in the world, including themselves, can reach the point of committing such atrocities. Young people need to understand the stages of the process that leads to mass executions and what the early warning signs of that process are. Those lessons have already been incorporated in peace building and reconciliation programs. However, civic education, ethics, moral philosophy, and peace building are still too often the preserve of informal education programs only. There is a long way to go before they are incorporated in traditional, institutional history curricula.

Notes

1 Marija Farmer is the author of the script for the performance *Ta Tvoja Mund Harmonika* (2016), while the other three performances were based on similar concepts and inspiration from the training and were directed by training participants: *Sjenka Duše* (2016, independently directed by Dragana Miljković), *Mi Smo Preostali* (2017, directed by Timka Omanović, with supervision by Marija Farmer), and *Žute Čizme* (2018, directed by Alen Osmić).
2 At this point I owe a brief explanation on visiting Vilina Vlas as a former "rape hotel," as the reader could also be disturbed and as visiting this place demands its own full analytical attention. For this purpose, I am writing a separate piece on so called in-situ learning that problematizes in more detail the question of memory sites and sites that were places of atrocities but which restarted their services after the war.
3 The Sarajevo-based NGO Post-Conflict Research Centre partnered with US-based Art of Revolution to establish the project for the 20th Commemoration of the Genocide in Srebrenica. This project previously brought together over 2,500 volunteers from

across the United States to lay out 1,000,000 handcrafted bones in the National Mall in Washington, DC, as a visible protest against ongoing genocide and mass atrocities occurring around the world. For more, see http://www.onemillionbones.net/ (retrieved: 7 January 2019).

4 Paraphrasing the term used for discussing the "dark tourism" in Auschwitz, available at http://bocktherobber.com/2013/10/has-auschwitz-become-the-disneyland-of-misery/.

5 For a full elaboration of a comparsion of Stanton's model in the case of genocidal war rapes in Bosnia and Herzegovina, refer to N. Močnik, "Sexual abuse of Muslim women in Balkan conflict in 1990s and the question of the hidden genocide," in *Islam in the Balkans: From Times of Glory to Times of Humility*, ed. Muhammet Savaş Kafkasyali (Ankara: T.C. Başbakanlık Türk İşbirliği ve Koordinasyon Ajansı Başkanlığı, 2016), 397–431.

6 See, for instance, projects run by Pro-Bodućnost (https://probuducnost.ba/), TPO Foundation (www.tpo.ba), Most Mira (www.mostmiraproject.org), and Centar za izgradnju mira (www.unvocim.net).

Bibliography

Ahonen, S. 2012. *Coming to terms with a dark past. How post-conflict societies deal with history*. Frankfurt: Peter Lang.

Ahonen, S. 2014. "Education in post-conflict societies." *Historical Encounters* 1 (1): 75–87.

Akman, K. B. 2015. "Sociotherapy as a contemporary alternative." *Bangladesh E-Journal of Sociology* 12 (1): 9–16.

Asavei, M. A. 2019. "The art and politics of imagination: Remembering mass violence against women." *Critical Review of International Social and Political Philosophy*. 22 (5): 618–636. doi: 10.1080/13698230.2019.1565704.

Auerbach, Y. 2009. "The reconciliation pyramid: A narrative based framework for analysing identity conflicts." *Political Psychology* 30 (2): 291–318.

Auerhahn, N. and Laub, D. 1998. "The primal scene of atrocity: The dynamic interplay between knowledge and fantasy of the Holocaust in children of survivors." *Psychoanalytic Psychology* 15 (3): 360–377.

Bajramović, S. 2018. *Hierarchical sisterhood. Supporting women's peacebuilding through Swedish aid to Bosnia-Herzegovina 1993–2013*. Örebro: Örebro University Print.

Bal, M. 2001. *Looking in: The art of viewing*. Amsterdam: Gordon and Breach.

Bar-On, D. 1999. *The indescribable and the undiscussable: Reconstructing human discourse after trauma*. Budapest, Hungary: Central European University Press.

Bar-On, D. 2006. *Tell your life story: Creating dialogue among Jews and Germans, Israelis and Palestinians*. Budapest: Central European University Press.

Barry, K. 1979. *Female sexual slavery*. Englewood Cliffs, NJ: Prentice-Hall.

Bekerman, Z. and Zembylas, M. 2011. *Teaching contested narratives: Identity, memory and reconciliation in peace education and beyond*. New York: Cambridge University Press.

Berry, M. E. 2017. "Barriers to women's progress after atrocity: Evidence from Rwanda and Bosnia–Herzegovina." *Gender and Society* 31 (6): 830–853.

Bertaux, D. and Thompson, P. 2005. "Introduction." In D. Bertaux and P. Thompson (Eds.), *Between generations: Family models, myths and memories* (2–12). New Jersey: Transaction Publishers.

Bieber, F. 2002. "Aid dependency in Bosnian politics and civil society: Failures and successes of post-war peacebuilding in Bosnia–Herzegovina." *Croatian International Relations Review* 8 (26): 25–29.

Brock-Utne, B. 1985. *Educating for peace: A feminist perspective.* New York: Pergamon Press.

Bloomfield, D. 2006. *On good terms: Clarifying reconciliation.* Berlin: Berghoff Foundation.

Brown, M., Boege, V., Clements, K., and Nolan, A. 2010. "Challenging state-building as peacebuilding: Working with hybrid political orders to build peace." In O. Richmond (Ed.), *Palgrave advances in peacebuilding: Critical developments and approaches* (99–115). London: Palgrave.

Burt, M. R. 1980. "Cultural myths and supports for rape." *Journal of Personality and Social Psychology* 38 (2): 217–230.

Clark, N. J. 2016. "Working with survivors of war rape and sexual violence fieldwork reflections from Bosnia–Hercegovina." *Qualitative Research* 17 (4): 424–439.

Cole, E. A. and Barsalou, J. 2006. *Unite or divide? The challenges of teaching history in societies emerging from violent conflict.* Washington, DC: United States Institute of Peace.

Crocker, J., Major, B., and Steele, C. 1998. "Social stigma." In D. T. Gilbert and S. T. Fiske (Eds.), *The handbook of social psychology* (504–553). Boston, MA: McGraw-Hill.

D'Adamo, L. and Fallace, T. 2011. "The multigenre research project: An approach to developing historical approach." *Social Studies Research and Practice* 6 (1): 75–88.

Das, V. 2007. *Life and words. Violence and the descent into the ordinary.* Oakland: University of California Press.

Davis, O., Yeager, E., and Foster, S. (Eds.). 2001. *Historical empathy and perspective taking in the social studies.* New York: Rowman and Littlefield.

Davies, W. 2016. *The happiness industry: How the government and big business sold us wellbeing.* London: Verso.

Davies, W. 2017. "On mental health, the royal family is doing more than our government." Available at https://www.theguardian.com/commentisfree/2017/apr/20/mental-health-royal-family-government-children-illness (accessed 8 March 2019).

Delić, A. and Avdibegović, E. 2016. "Shame and silence in the aftermath of war rape in Bosnia and Herzegovina: 22 years later." Available at https://www.researchgate.net/p ublication/293 815848_Shame_and_Silence_in_the_aftermath_of_War_Rape_in_Bos nia_and_Herzegovina_22_years_later (accessed 9 March 2019).

Eastmond, M. 2010. "Reconciliation, reconstruction and everyday life in war torn societies." *Focaal: Journal of Global and Historical Anthropology* 57: 3–16.

Edelson, M. 1970. *Sociotherapy and psychotherapy.* Chicago: University of Chicago Press.

Francis, D. 2002. *People, peace and power: Conflict transformation in action.* London: Pluto Press.

Freire, P. 1970. *Pedagogy of the oppressed.* New York: Herder and Herder.

Funk, J. and Good, N. 2017. *Neizlječena trauma: Rad na ozdravljenju I izgradnji mira u BiH.* Sarajevo: TPO Fondacija.

Gavey, N. 2005. *Just sex: The cultural scaffolding of rape.* Hove and Brighton: Routledge.

Goffman, E. 1963. *Stigma: Notes on the management of spoiled identity.* Harmondsworth: Penguin Books.

Halilovich, H. 2015. "Long-distance mourning and synchronised memories in a global context: Commemorating Srebrenica in diaspora." *Journal of Muslim Minority Affairs* 35 (3): 410–422.

Helms, E. 2014. "Rejecting Angelina: Bosnian war rape survivors and the ambiguities of sex in war." *Slavic Review* 73 (3): 612–634.

Hesford, W. S. 1999. "Reading 'rape stories': Material rhetoric and the trauma of representation." *College English* 62 (2): 1992–221.

Hirsch, M. 2012. *The Generation of postmemory: Writing and visual culture after the Holocaust.* New York: Columbia University Press.

Hoogenbom, D. and Vieille, S. 2010. "Rebuilding social fabric in failed states: Examining transitional justice in Bosnia." *Human Rights Review* 11 (2): 183–198.

Husić, S., Šiljak, I., Osmanović, E., Đekić, F., and Heremić, L. 2014. *Još uvijek smo žive! Istraživanje o dugoročnim posljedicama ratnog silovanja i strategijama suočavanja preživjelih u Bosni i Hercegovini.* Medica: Zenica.

Igreja, V. 2008. "Memories as qeapons: The politics of peace and silence in post-civil war Mozambique." *Journal of Southern African Studies* 34 (3): 539–556.

Israfilova, F. and Khoo-Lattimore, C. 2018. "Sad and violent but I enjoy it: Children's engagement with dark tourism as an educational tool." *Tourism and Hospitality Research* 1: 1–10.

Jacobs, J. 2016. "The memorial at Srebrenica: Gender and the social meanings of collective memory in Bosnia–Herzegovina." *Memory Studies* 10 (4): 423–439.

Jansen, S. 2013. "If reconciliation is the answer are we asking right questions?" *Studies in Social Justice* 7 (2): 229–243.

Jones, B., Jeffrey, A., and Jakala, M. 2012. "The 'transitional citizen': Civil society, political agency and hopes for transitional justice in Bosnia and Herzegovina." InO. Simićand Z. Volčić (Eds.), *Transitional Justice and Civil Society in the Balkans* (87–103). New York: Springer.

Josse, E. 2010. "'They came with two guns': The consequences of sexual violence for the mental health of women in armed conflicts." *International Review of the Red Cross* 92 (877): 177–195.

Kannenberg, R. L. 2003. *Sociotherapy for sociopaths – Resocial group.* Dublin: Premier Publishing.

Kaplan, L. 1996. *No voice is ever wholly lost. An exploration of the everlasting attachment between parent and child.* New York: Simon & Schuster.

Kappler, S. 2013. "Peacebuilding and lines of friction between imagined communities in Bosnia–Herzegovina and South Africa." *Peacebuilding* 1 (3): 349–364.

Karge, H. and Batarilo, K. 2008. "Reform in the field of history in education Bosnia and Herzegovina: Modernization of history textbooks in Bosnia and Herzegovina: From the withdrawal of offensive material from textbooks in 1999 to the new generation of textbooks in 2007/2008." Available at http://repository.gei.de/bitstream/handle/11428/264/Karge_Batarilo_Reform.pdf.

Kelly, L. 1988. *Surviving sexual violence.* New Jersey: Wiley.

Klein, E. 1998. "International aspects of the conflict in the Former Yugoslavia." In Y. Danieli (Ed.), *International handbook of multigenerational legacies of trauma* (279–295). New York: Plenum Press.

Knaus, G. and Martin, F. 2003. "Travails of the European Raj." *Journal of Democracy* 14 (3): 60–74.

Korostelina, K. 2013. *History education in the formation of social identity.* New York: Palgrave MacMillian.

Lederach, J. P. 1997. *Building peace: Sustainable reconciliation in divided societies.* Washington: Institute of Peace Press.

Lengel, L. 2018. "Mediated memory work and resistant remembering of wartime sexual violence, 1992–1995." *Feminist Media Studies* 18 (2): 325–328.

Link, B. and Phelan, J. 2014. "Stigma power." *Social Science and Medicine* 103: 24–32.

Lončar, M., Medvedev, V., Jovanović, N. and Hotujac, L. 2006. "Psychological consequences of rape on women in 1991–1995 war in Croatia and Bosnia and Herzegovina." *Croatian Medical Journal* 47 (1): 67–75.

Mandi, F. D., Williams, S. L., Rife, S. C., and Cantrell, P. 2015. "Examining cultural, social, and self-related aspects of stigma in relation to sexual assault and trauma symptoms." *Violence Against Women* 21 (5): 598–615.

Mannergren Selimovic, J. 2013. "Making peace, making memory: Peacebuilding and politics of remembrance at memorials of mass atrocities." *Peacebuilding Journal* 1 (3): 334–348.

Mannheim, K. 1972. "The problems of generations." In Karl Mannheim (Ed.), *Essays in the sociology of knowledge* (276–322). London: Routledge.

McCully, A. 2012. "History teaching, conflict and the legacy of the past." *Education, Citizenship and Social Justice* 7 (2): 145–159.

McGrattan, C. and Stephen Hopkins. 2016. "Memory in post-conflict societies: From contention to integration?" *Ethnopolitics* 16 (5): 488–499.

Mobekk, E. 2005. "Transitional justice in post-conflict societies. Approaches to reconciliation." In A. Ebnother and P. Fluri (Eds.), *After intervention: Public security management in post-conflict societies.* (261–292) Geneva: Geneva Centre for the Democratic Control of Armed Forces.

Murphy, K. and Gallagher, T. 2009. "Reconstruction after violence: How teachers and schools can deal with the legacy of the past." *Perspectives in Education* 27 (2): 11.

Nordquist, K. 2017. *Reconciliation as politics: A concept and its practice.* Eugene, OR: Pickwick Publications.

O'Reilly, M. 2012. "Muscular interventionism." *International Feminist Journal of Politics* 14 (4): 529–548.

Orford, A. 2003. *Reading humanitarian intervention: Human rights and the use of force in international law.* Cambridge: Cambridge University Press.

Parent, G. 2016. "Local peacebuilding, trauma, and empowerment in Bosnia–Herzegovina." *Peace and Change* 41 (4): 510–538.

Paris, R. 2004. *At war's end: Building peace after civil conflict.* Cambridge: Cambridge University Press.

Parker, R. and Aggleton, P. 2003. "HIV and AIDS-related stigma and discrimination: A conceptual framework and implications for action." *Social Science and Medicine* 57 (1) 13–24.

Pašalić-Kreso, A. 2008. "The war and post-war impact on the educational system of Bosnia and Herzegovina." *International Review of Education* 54 (3): 353–374.

Pavlowitch, S. K. 2004. "History education in the Balkans: How bad is it?" *Journal of Southern Europe and the Balkans* 6 (1): 63–68.

Pescosolido, B. and Martin, J. 2015. "The stigma complex." *Annual Review of Sociology* 41: 87–116.

Pilgrim, D. and McCranie, A. 2013. *Recovery and mental health: A critical sociological account.* Basingstoke, UK: Palgrave Macmillan.

Quinn, D. M. and Chaudoir, S. R. 2009. "Living with a concealable stigmatized identity: The impact of anticipated stigma, centrality, salience, and cultural stigma on psychological distress and health." *Journal of Personality and Social Psychology* 97: 634–651.

Richetrs, A., Rutayisire, T., and Dekker, C. 2010. "Care as a turning point in sociotherapy: Remaking the moral world in post-genocide Rwanda." *Medische Antropologie* 22 (1): 93–108.

Richmond, O. P. 2004. "The globalization of responses to conflict and the peacebuilding consensus." *Cooperation and Conflict* 39 (2): 129–150.

Sayce, L. 1998. "Stigma, discrimination and social exclusion: What's in a word." *Journal of Mental Health* 7 (4): 331–343.

Schaap, A. 2008. "Reconciliation as ideology and politics." *Constellations: An International Journal of Democratic and Critical Theory* 15 (2): 249–264.

Schank, R. C. 1990. *Tell me a story: A new look at real and artificial memory.* New York: Macmillan.

Simić, O. 2009. "What remains of Srebrenica? Motherhood, transitional justice and yearning for the truth." *Journal of International Women's Studies* 10 (4): 220–236.

Simić, O. 2018. *Silenced victims of wartime sexual violence.* New York: Routledge.

Simić, O. and Volčić, Z. 2014. "In the land of wartime rape: Bosnia, cinema and reparation." *Griffith Journal of Law and Human Dignity* 2 (2): 377–401.

Skjelsbaek, I. 2006. "Therapeutic work with victims of sexual violence in war and postwar: A discourse analysis of Bosnian experiences." *Peace and Conflict Journal of Peace Psychology* 12 (2): 93–118.

Smith, A. 2011. *Education and peacebuilding: From "conflict-analysis" to "conflict transformation"?* Retrieved from http://uir.ulster.ac.uk/19794/ (accessed 27 February 2019).

Smart, L. and Wegner, D. 1999. "Covering up what can't be seen: Concealable stigma and mental control." *Journal of Personality and Social Psychology* 77 (3): 474–486.

Solga, K. 2006. "Rape's metatheatrical return: Rehearsing sexual violence among the early moderns." *Theatre Journal* 58 (1): 53–72.

Stiglmayer, A. 1994. "The war in the Former Yugoslavia." In A. Stiglmayer (Ed.), *Mass rape: The war against women in Bosnia–Herzegovina* (1–34). Lincoln: University of Nebraska Press.

Thaler, M. 2018. *Naming violence: A critical theory of genocide, torture, and terrorism.* New York: Columbia University Press.

Tyler, I. 2013. *Revolting subjects: Social abjection and resistance in neoliberal Britain.* London: Zed.

Tyler, I. and Slater, T. 2018. "Rethinking the sociology of stigma." *The Sociological Review Monographs* 66 (4): 721–743.

UN. 2017. "Shame, stigma integral to logic of sexual violence as war tactic, special adviser tells security council, as speakers demand recognition for survivors." Available at https://www.un.org/press/en/2017/sc12819.doc.htm (accessed 8 March 2019).

Vinitzky-Seroussi, V. and Teeger, C. 2010. "Unpacking the unspoken: Silence in collective memory and forgetting." *Social Forces* 88 (3): 1103–1122.

Wacquant, L. 2008. *Urban outcasts: A comparative sociology of advanced marginality.* Cambridge: Polity.

Whiteley, J. S. 1986. "Sociotherapy and psychotherapy in the treatment of personality disorder: Discussion paper." *Journal of the Royal Society of Medicine* 79: 721–725.

Winter, J. 2010. "Thinking about silence." In E. Ben-Zeev, R. Ginio, and J. Winter (Eds.), *Shadows of war: A social history of silence in the twentieth century* (3–31). New York: Cambridge University Press.

World Vision. 2016. *No shame in justice addressing stigma against survivors to end sexual violence in conflict zones.* Available at https://assets.worldvision.org.uk/files/7214/5806/4579/Stigma_Summary_Report.pdf (accessed 9 March 2019).

Yordanova, K. 2015. "The second generation's imagery of the Bosnian war (1992–1995)." *Anthropology of East Europe Review* 33 (1): 70–86.

7 Survivors and postwar youth in intergenerational dialogue to prevent the transmission of sexual traumas

Women in politically unstable or conflict-affected patriarchal societies are exposed to rapes and unwanted pregnancies, and reportedly experience severe, potentially lifelong trauma. Traumatized mothers – survivors of collective violence fleeing from their homes due to the conflict or as a result of witnessing extreme violence – can furthermore put their children at risk of developing maladaptive and asocial behaviors through transmission of their trauma. Despite the traumatizing impact that chaotic sociopolitical events have on mothers, in many cultural contexts these women are furthermore expected to prioritize the well-being and/or survival of their children before sufficiently taking care of themselves. While they remain pillars of their households in patriarchal societies around the globe, they also face the extraordinary social pressure of being responsible to raise their offspring. At the same time, they are the first to be blamed for failing to break the cycles of violence that are presumably perpetuated through transmitted collective trauma.

Throughout this book, I have stressed the importance of moving away from the prevailing therapeutic and clinical understanding of trauma – an understanding that, directly or not, puts pressure and full responsibility on the traumatized individuals when it comes to healing and recovery in the aftermath of war. That one might be transmitting trauma to future generations could be interpreted by survivors as a lack of control over their own trauma and/or their failure to heal from it or successfully cope with it. There are a number of ways in which the traumas of survivors of war rape are approached well into the aftermath of the conflict by important social agents, among which I include peace educators, impact ideas, perceptions, behavioral patterns, and understandings of (violent) cultural scripts of sexuality, naturalized gender-based violence, and support for the toxic aspects of the patriarchal social order. The narrated silences and underaddressed topics of sexual violence in peace education and in critical history teaching are two examples of such support. I therefore propose that the traumatic legacy of women survivors of war rape should be studied within the power structures of cultural patterns, inflicted primarily by society, which threaten the future security of entire communities and which manifest not only as a collective memory but also as a contributor to the continued cultural patterns that shape our understanding of sexuality and gender.

I embarked upon this research with the intention of providing a context-specific understanding of the complex nexus at which women survivors of war-related sexual crimes (now mothers) and the risks for transmitting trauma in the context of family upbringing collaborate to perpetuate ethnic division, intergroup hatred, and mistrust in postconflict Bosnia-Herzegovina. As an educator, my main motivation was to examine family relations and the toxic environments that produced the youth with whom we work. I started with the premise, based on previous scholarship, that subconscious transmission, which is usually manifested in silence and the suppression of traumatic memory and PTSD symptoms, might prevent these youth from establishing relationships that promote postconflict mutual coexistence, respect for stories from the "other side," compassion and caring for others, and shared responsibility for the future of the whole community. Trauma transmission from mother–survivors of war rapes invades the spheres of the private and the intimate, and risks shattering existing intergenerational dynamics by exposing youth to what the family has so far attempted to protect them from pain, rage, and sometimes hatred. As I am largely unfamiliar with the ways in which youth respond to parental trauma, and to avoid the risk of negatively impacting their social dynamics, I decided to limit the scope of this research primarily to the mothers' perspectives and understanding of trauma transmission and the legacy of war rape. However, I look forward to how this collected knowledge can inform and further my practice as a teacher in the field of peace education and sexual violence prevention.

As for the frequently expressed fears among mothers that sharing their traumatic pasts will necessarily transfer their trauma, I believe that these fears are the result of a lack of spaces (both metaphorical and physical) and instruction that could prepare both the teller and the receiver for sharing and also help to explain why this sharing is important. Dismantling the stubborn systems of trauma narratives must involve the systematic and intentional creation of spaces and methods where mothers can learn how to share and youth can learn how to witness and process these traumatic stories. While this would be best as a part of formal postconflict education, I am also aware that schools as state-controlled institutions are the hardest to change when it comes to critical peace education. But learning never happens in complete isolation: information and knowledge transmission occur *before*, *after*, and outside the school, through family, religious institutions, popular culture, and social media. As opposed to state institutions and formal education, which employ a national, official explanation for historical "truths," educating outside of these ideologically driven spaces is much wilder, demanding that the educator reflect critically on her own personal narratives and experiences – especially if she survived and/or witnessed the conflict herself. She must confront her own biases and assumptions and take an honest position with regard to the mainstream historical narratives and those who surround her and impact her psychosocial background.

In addition, the practice of learning in such contexts extends toward mediating and, as the process also addresses the students' emotional triggers and (post) traumatic stress, sometimes counseling. Reflecting on the teaching of war-rape and sexual violence legacies is, as with any other (history) class that covers the recent violent conflict, complex, sensitive, and emotionally exhausting for both teacher and student, especially if such education is undertaken in a fragile region that has not yet come to terms with their traumatic pasts. If prepared thoughtfully and carefully, however, such education carries important reconciliatory potential that can have long-term impact on the lives of individuals. On this subject I disagree with Bar-On and Card, who claim that some crimes and atrocities are simply indescribable, that there is no language capable of capturing such horrific experiences. But the traumatic experience lacks a language only if the burden to communicate the trauma continues to fall on the survivors. As soon as we start speaking of collective traumas, the language necessary for it is provided in the first- or secondhand experiences and ideas that are shared among community members. For us as a society, the learning moment occurs not in the language created only by survivors, but by everyone who passively or actively takes part in this process – as a fellow survivor, a co-healer, a witness, a co-creator, a consumer, or a user.

A woman who has never articulated her own traumatic experiences, but who joins a sharing circle to listen to others, creates her own language of this (same) trauma. Language – or an intergenerational physical and metaphorical space(s) of trauma sharing – is therefore no longer owned solely by the survivors, but by all social actors. I believe that these various experiences, bodies of knowledge, and backgrounds can only help to break the one-way transmission of trauma from survivors to youth. The risk of transmitting what we can define as the destructive and toxic intergenerational effects of trauma – manifested in intergroup hatred and/or revenge fantasies – exists only when survivors insist on retaining ownership of their traumatic experiences, as survivors believe that only they can really describe the pain, the long-term legacy, and tell the truth. The therapeutic approach to healing trauma helps to deepen this feeling of ownership, as the survivor is either left alone in the process of her healing or is surrounded only by fellow survivors – that is, only those who experienced the same trauma can understand her. This approach, which sees survivors as an isolated island, does not invite the participation of other social members, including their families.

For the youth, it creates a narrative that this was not "their war." This presents a contradiction, because there is simultaneously social pressure on these youth – often institutionalized in history curricula – to remember this same war and to keep its memory alive even when the survivors have passed away. If there is no language to describe the atrocities, it is because we are waiting for the survivors to create it; and the survivors, while not finding it themselves, at the same time reject the interpretations of others, perceiving anyone but the survivor merely as a passive witness, a listener. But if the language of survivors is to be understood by their audience – their descendants – it must use metaphorical signs and symbols that are used and recognized by the same audience. These signs and symbols must be understandable to those who did not experience and/or witness those atrocities. Rather than thinking of the transmission of trauma as a passive process that must preoccupy survivors – particularly as it relates to preventing it or transmitting only non-toxic memories – it should be considered a dialogical process of mutual exchange that can have both preventive and rehabilitation benefits.

Traumatic experiences and PTSD symptoms are medicalized, meaning that one eventually strives to be rid of them, to ultimately move on with a life that is free of trauma. However, intergenerational dialogue might challenge this idea of desirable and definite closure and instead help to transform the traumatic legacy. An intergenerational exchange between survivors and postwar youth would give the youth access to very personal and intimate accounts of the war – information that might be lacking, for example, in media coverage. This same exchange might help survivors reintegrate into the broader society, forcing them out of their comfortable but closed circles of fellow survivors and enabling them to assume a social role other than that of "survivor." However, this dialogue can only transpire if survivors relinquish part of the ownership of their own experiences and testimonies, allowing the new generation to contextualize and interpret them from the perspective of those who, while they did not experience the atrocities first hand, must nevertheless live with their legacy. Survivors claim a desire for agency in their testimonies; in the aftermath of war, youth also reclaim agency for their own future. This includes their agendas as to how the war will take a constitutive part in this future.

In addition to their fear of transmitting the destructive effects of trauma, mother–survivors also emphasize that sharing their testimonies with their children and the postwar generations in general is important for the sake of imparting "historical lessons": learning how to prevent these same atrocities from ever happening again. But while sharing personal experience can have a very powerful pedagogical effect, it can also be tricky when we think in terms of epistemological developments, particularly in the field of gender and sexuality. As our understanding of sexuality and gender has changed dramatically in the last few decades, the personal experiences of older generations do not necessarily fulfill the needs of their descendants. For example, while survivors will acknowledge the toxic nature of the patriarchal order that led to the wartime use of mass rapes, they would not necessarily see that this same order creates controlled patterns over diverse forms of sexuality. The experience of war rape makes survivors sometimes to believe to be more knowledgeable, informed and aware on toxic sexualities.

However, due to their background and strong social surroundings that remain mainly patriarchal, they might anyway not be able to acknowledge diverse, non-heterosexual sexualities, or the gender spectrum that goes beyond female and male, just to give an example. In addition, my simultaneous work with both survivors and youth has confirmed that the sexual and gender issues faced by these two generations might be very different; for instance, one of the main problems that we address in today's sexual violence prevention programs is digital sexual violence. This was not, and will not be, a concern for survivors. These generational clashes, which are manifested in knowledge and information gaps, make us realize that older generations are no longer the sole or even primary reference for youth education. What if youth resistance to remembrance or witnessing the testimonies of survivors is in fact a resistance to something that youth perceive as toxic, something they in fact want to forget? What if they are sufficiently knowledgeable and informed but simply want their own chance to start from scratch?

The memory culture of war-rape survivors today consists of narrated silences, blaming the victim, and nurturing the impunity of crimes through the stigmatization of survivors. If there are no social repercussions for the perpetrators of these crimes, but instead continuous symbolic punishment for survivors, how does this teach anyone that sexual violence is wrong? If working with trauma in the aftermath of conflict comprises rehabilitation processes in which survivors are responsible for their own healing, absent any other social members, how does this teach us that rape is not about individuals but about culture? None of these really teaches us how not to repeat toxic patterns; on the contrary, they all function as supportive mechanisms.

At the very least, what the existing memory culture of war-rape survivors calls for is a more systematic approach to ethnographic research and rehabilitation work with the so-called Other side – those generally considered perpetrators. In the context of the legacy of war rape, these are primarily boys and men. Due to a lack of knowledge, I often find myself feeling powerless and ineffectual when trying to think what to offer boys during sexual violence prevention workshops. These workshops attract and actively engage mostly girls, while boys too often respond defensively, or even with bullying, when presented with the testimonies of war-rape survivors. It is also very challenging, if not impossible, to reflect on the "Other" side with survivors and their families; husbands and older male family members do not usually talk much about them. Their sons reject any connection to or relation with "men as perpetrators," even though they often generalize about the male population in their own communities. Survivors easily see mothers from "the other side" as bearing responsibility and blame for raising the perpetrators; however, they would never see themselves doing the same.

Nurturing forgiveness and empathy (mothers to mothers, for instance) in such a context proved extremely difficult for most of the mothers, posing a great challenge to peace educators for whom empathy and forgiveness are crucial components in achieving peace and reconciliation. When women survivors contextualize survivors from "the other" group within their broader context, in which their male counterparts were (potentially) rapists and perpetrators, the results are often fear, mistrust, and sometime hate, with mothers blaming other mothers for bad mothering. Mothers who continue to grieve for their lost sons, or those who fear that they will raise their children with hatred as a result of their own trauma, might easily become intolerant to other social (ethnoreligious) groups. As opposed to conventional wisdom, in which the experiences of motherhood during wartime – sending their sons to the front, witnessing the murder of loved ones, seeing their daughters held captive – would presumably evoke a empathic connection and help rehumanize everyone involved in the conflict, this experience does not seem to ultimately connect mothers in developing relationships.

While mothers in a postconflict patriarchal context might all fight for the best future for their children, this does not presuppose the feminist agenda of a united struggle against sexism and militarism. It therefore suits the patriarchal society to portray mothers as peace workers, like the mothers of Srebrenica: while they mourn for their lost sons, husbands, and fathers, they do not challenge the system that allowed this to happen. On the other hand, feminists, particularly those anti-war and anti-military activists from the 1990s who gathered in protest against the war, do not frame their fight as a fight for their children but as a struggle against militarism and its necessary intersection with the broader oppression of women. A relatively new narrative has emerged through the strong presence of the Forgotten Children of War Association, which depicts war survivors – particularly those who gave birth as a result of rape – as heroines. They are considered such not only because of what they endured, but mostly due to the strength they have shown in fighting against stigma and social ostracism in the aftermath of the war. This narrative comes from the children, now young adults, and addresses the same audience. It is against forgetting, but in favor of forgiving and moving forward with their lives.

All of these narratives, although extremely important and compelling, are insufficient when it comes to transforming and changing the cultural patterns of sexuality and gender. While addressing the "other side" might target the mothers of oppressors, the testimonies of men – particularly those actively involved and whom we today define and understand as perpetrators – are missing. Until mothers are able to think of their sons as possible perpetrators, which would mean that they are able to recognize the cultural patterns that lead one to commit violence, it is impossible to design effective reconciliatory policies. Mothers who are aware of the violent actions of their sons, husbands, brothers, and fathers will rarely see these actions as crimes because it is never a crime when a man acts to protect himself or his family. At the same time, it is hard to see the men from the other side as protectors. They are almost always occupiers, and yes, criminals. But if survivors strongly believe that the next generation must learn from the past to avoid repeating the crime, is it not possible that we can also learn from the perpetrators? For instance, can individuals like Esad Landžo contribute to peace education and sexual violence prevention programs? If so, how?

We have very insufficient evidence as to how perpetrators "recover in the aftermath of war," which helps to sustain the survivors' image of the perpetrators as they remember it from the war: the rapists, the murderers, the aggressors. There is recognition of the survivor who succeeds in finding ways to cope with her trauma and seeks reintegration with society as an equal member, but there is no such social acknowledgment for the perpetrators. Moreover, what remains truly unspeakable today is not the survivors' trauma and its painful legacy, but the fact that the perpetrators are members of our families – as fathers, as family breeders. As long as peace education and "learning from the past" rely primarily on the legacy of sexual violence or solely on the testimonies of survivors, we will keep failing to see sexual violence as a system of relations and dynamics; instead, we will continue to divide people – men as perpetrators, women as victims – according to traditional understandings of binary gender roles.

With that said, I would like to emphasize once again that I am aware of diverse and complex gender role dynamics as they relate to sexual violence in war, and that I do not assume that women are only victims and men are only perpetrators. I am also aware of earlier postwar scholarship that warned of dangerous essentialist writings which ignored the many men who were subjected to sexual violence, or the numerous women who participated equally in combat and in the general aggression committed against others. Nor am I limiting all sexual relationships in the aftermath of the war to heterosexual ones that are not subjected to sexist and patriarchal norms. However, although I am aware of all this diversity and its rich expressions among individuals, most of my ethnographic data were collected in a traditional, heterosexual context with clearly defined and limited ideas of binary, essentialist gender roles – both in peace and war. This became particularly important when I had the chance to work with two generations – one comprising survivors (around 55–60 years old) and one comprising postwar youth (around 15–17 years old).

As a peace worker who emphasizes the prevention of sexual violence, the emergence of new knowledge and information that resulted from the meeting of these two generations is very exciting, providing "this something" that we can learn from history. When the generation of survivors shares their collective memories with those who have not experienced such violence – allowing those memories to be openly interpreted, altered, and used in the context of postwar generations – the trauma transmission is no longer a haunting legacy that nurtures revenge fantasies that necessarily lead to a destructive future. Instead of trying to suppress these memories with silence and fear, a mutual dialogue of open sharing can become truly rehabilitative for survivors and preventive for postwar generations. Considered to be safe spaces, the associations for war-rape survivors were presumably places of trauma-healing and empowerment in which survivors could regain control over their lives, reclaim certain social roles (for instance, that of the mother), and thus reintegrate in social life. Such therapeutic support circles, where survivors meet fellow survivors, have helped a significant number of women recover and make progress in their journey of healing from trauma.

However, these same circles became at a certain point something like "nurseries" for the collective trauma. While their closeness and repetitive narratives helped one deal with PTSD symptoms, they were not necessarily *reconciliatory*. Those circles are de facto very monolithic: survivors built these comforts zones without meeting other individuals from their environment, whether cross-generationally, cross-ethnically, cross-religiously, or cross-gender. This limits the mothers' healing practice in dealing with the legacy of war rapes to their own internalized experience. In the aftermath of the war, they must deal with the intersection of complex, potentially violent and abusive social dynamics that divide along both ethnoreligious and sexuality-gender lines. Most of the mothers in the peripheral regions where I conducted the majority of my ethnographic research apply traditional hegemonic patriarchal rules to their mothering practice, exchanging their mothering practices primarily in this kind of closed circle.

It is therefore not trauma as such that can be dangerous when transmitted from survivors to their offspring. What I believe is truly dangerous, and which disables an effective reconciliation process that could engage postwar youth, is that the circles of survivors (and perpetrators, I assume) are very clearly divided: the work that challenges the stigma against survivors is still to be found mainly in the domain of the survivors themselves and in organizations that deal with gender and women's issues. This is what keeps "historical trauma" alive and perpetuated in succeeding generations. The absence of active exchange among different social groups supports the social perception that gender-based violence is a women's issue and that the stigma associated with sexual violence is the survivors' burden. I believe that the knowledge and information collected from mother–survivors must be incorporated more broadly into peace programs and must address young people cross-generationally, cross-ethnically, cross-religiously, cross-gender, and beyond. However, the exchange must flow in both directions: survivors today have much to learn from those who never experienced the war.

Index

Printed in the United States
by Baker & Taylor Publisher Services

Printed in the United States
by Baker & Taylor Publisher Services